UNSTOPPABLE
AFTER 40

THE SECRETS TO AVOIDING INJURY, SUPERCHARGING ENERGY, AND NEVER SLOWING DOWN

BY **MILO F. BRYANT, CSCS** AND THE EDITORS OF **Men'sHealth**

This book is intended as a reference volume only, not as a medical manual. The information given here is designed to help you make informed decisions about your health. It is not intended as a substitute for any treatment that may have been prescribed by your doctor. If you suspect that you have a medical problem, we urge you to seek competent medical help.

Mention of specific companies, organizations, or authorities in this book does not imply endorsement by the author or publisher, nor does mention of specific companies, organizations, or authorities imply that they endorse this book, its author, or the publisher.

Book design by Made Visible Studio

Cover Photography by PeopleImages/E+ via Getty Images

Interior Photography: Getty Images: dima_sidelnikov/iStock/Getty Images Plus: 40; Dziggyfoto/iStock/Getty Images Plus: 4-5; Eva-Katalin/E+: 26; grinvalds/iStock/Getty Images Plus: 34; G-Stock Faces/iStock/Getty Images Plus: 28; Image Source/Image Source: 32; Juan Moyano/Moment: 90; Klaus Vedfelt/DigitalVision: 11; Kolostock: 88; Marco_Piunti/E+: 96; mihailomilovanovic/E+: 29; miniseries/E+: 23; Moof/Image Source: 19; Nomad/E+: 27; PeopleImages/E+: 30, 95; PM Images/Stone: 102; SolStock/E+: 21; Suradech14/iStock/Getty Images Plus: 14; svetikd/E+: 16; Tara Moore/Stone: 42; The Good Brigade/DigitalVision: 3; Thomas Barwick/DigitalVision: 13; Thomas Barwick/DigitalVision: 17; Vladimir Gnedin/iStock/Getty Images Plus: 37; Westend61/E+: 8, 65; Anna Efetova/Moment: 92; triloks/E+: 24; Brian Kim: 7

Illustrations by Kyle Hilton

Library of Congress Cataloging-in-Publication Data is on file with the publisher.

ISBN 978-1-955710-03-9

Printed in China

2 4 6 8 10 9 7 5 3 1 paperback

HEARST

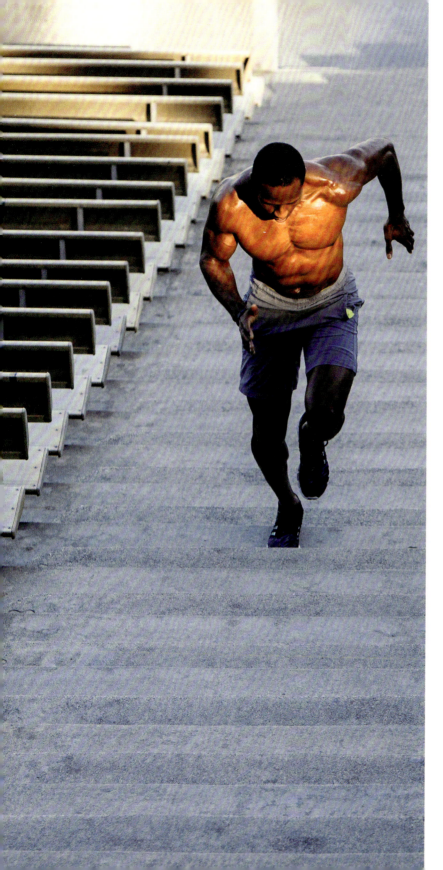

MH
UNSTOPPABLE AFTER 40

TABLE OF CONTENTS

THE WARMUP

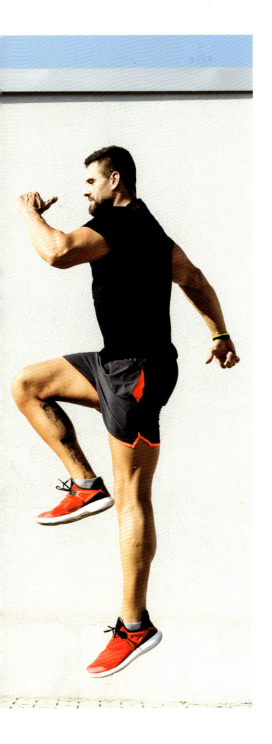

THE COOLDOWN

BULLETPROOF TOTAL BODY SERIES

INTRODUCTION

I HAVEN'T always been a full-time professional fitness trainer, but I can remember the exact moment I wanted to become one.

In 2006, I was working for the *Colorado Springs Gazette*, writing two columns: one about sports and one about physical fitness. Each summer, the newspaper ran a Fitness Challenge program, where one person would receive three months of free fitness training from me, and we would chronicle their weight loss transformation, complete with before and after pictures.

People would write, email, fax, or snail mail me a 300-word letter detailing why I should choose them, agreeing to publicly disclose their height, weight, body fat percentage, and more. That year, I chose Ted: a 66-year-old man with type 2 diabetes. Ted was obese and had high blood pressure and a pacemaker; he'd also had a hip replacement three months before we met. He was taking too many medications to list.

From a health standpoint, Ted was in horrible shape. But like many of us, he wanted to put more life into the years he had left. And there was one way in particular he wanted to do that.

"Can you train me to play pain-free golf?" he asked me.

The *Gazette* chronicled Ted's journey over the next three months. Not just the workouts, but the victories and defeats, too.

Then one mid-August day, Ted and I teed off at the Country Club of Colorado. My first shot went in the bushes; his was short, but down the middle of the fairway. I hit into some weeds behind the green, while he hit to just in front of the green. Ted then chipped to within five feet. I hacked out next, still 30 feet from the hole. Ted lined up his putt. Addressed the ball. Smooth stroke back, smooth stroke through the ball.

Par.

Ted bent over and reached his hand into the cup. As he started to stand up, he hesitated. My anxiety set in; I thought something was wrong. Ted took off his glasses and wiped tears from his eyes. Then he hugged me.

I stood there, dumbfounded, as Ted whispered in my ear, "I couldn't do this last year. I couldn't even do this six months ago. I'd putt, and my wife had to pick up the ball for me. I couldn't even pick up my own putt. Thank you, thank you, thank you. You've given me back my life."

If you're like most older guys, then you might have the same goal Ted did—all you want to do is enjoy the activities you love pain-free. Maybe that's going on long runs, lifting heavy weights in the gym, or just keeping up with your kids during a game of backyard tag. After meeting Ted, I realized that all of us will have a similar goal—because we're all getting older. That's why I stopped writing about fitness and started training. Much of that training focused on guys like you, who lead busy lives and don't want to slow down just because they've added more candles to their birthday cake.

With this book, I hope to give you the tools to move with more energy and less pain. To feel your best at 40 and beyond. Whether you want to recover faster from your workouts or simply avoid busting your back on the golf course, I will show you how to become unstoppable in everything you do.

Let's get started.

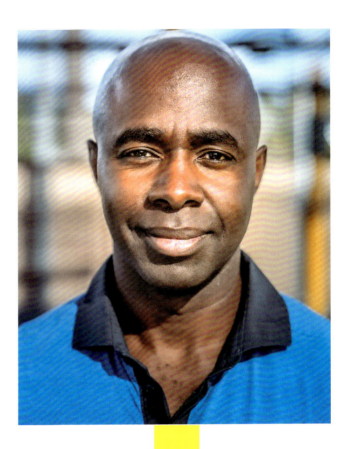

MEET YOUR COACH

MILO F. BRYANT, 50, CSCS, is a fitness coach, life coach, and the co-author of *Movement, Functional Movement Systems: Screening, Assessment, Corrective Strategies.* An athlete since childhood, he was 8 years old the first time he lied about his age and snuck into a weight room (sorry, Mom). Bryant specializes in training athletes for sports. His gym, called The Playground, is an entirely outdoor facility that encompasses 7,000 square feet in Del Mar, California. You can find him and his athletes flipping tractor tires, pulling sleds, and playing Hooverball as well as doing all the traditional lifts. Check him out at **MiloStrong.com.**

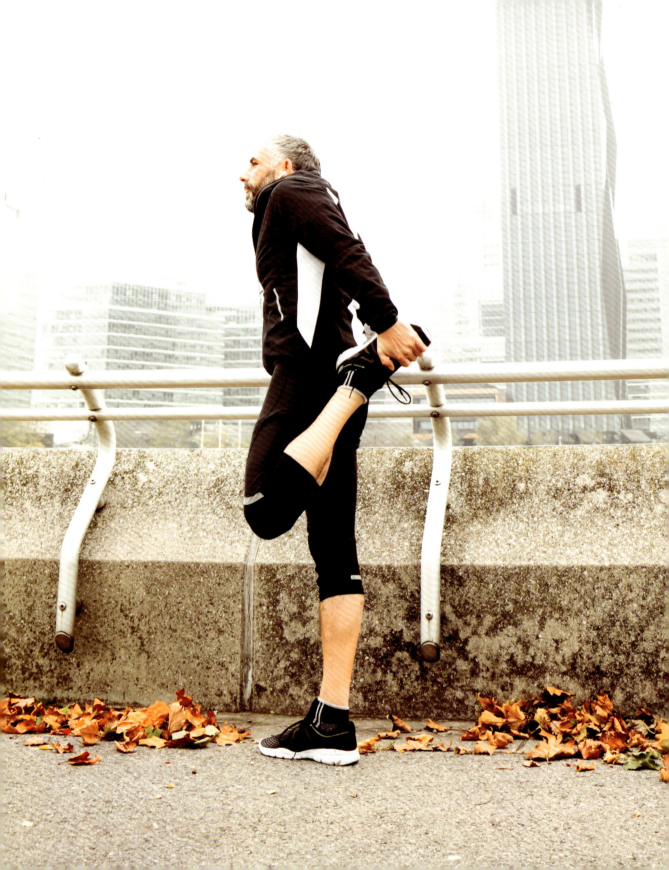

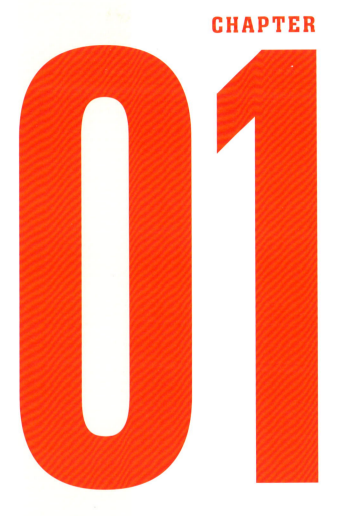

01

MEET YOUR BODY
AFTER 40

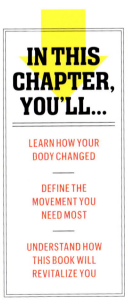

IN THIS CHAPTER, YOU'LL...

LEARN HOW YOUR
BODY CHANGED

—

DEFINE THE
MOVEMENT YOU
NEED MOST

—

UNDERSTAND HOW
THIS BOOK WILL
REVITALIZE YOU

YOUR BODY AFTER 40

BY THE NUMBERS

1-3%

HOW MUCH MUSCLE STRENGTH AND SIZE YOU LOSE EACH DECADE (STARTING AROUND AGE 50!)

1%

THE RATE AT WHICH YOUR CARDIO-VASCULAR ENDURANCE DECREASES EACH YEAR

5%

THE RATE AT WHICH YOUR METAB-OLISM SLOWS DOWN EACH DECADE AFTER AGE 40

YOU ARE not the same person at 40 as you were at 20. Be thankful! For the vast majority of us, that's a good thing.

Sure, after 40, you may ache a little more, and you may never bench as much as you did two decades ago—but you've also gained half a lifetime's worth of knowledge and memories.

In my opinion, the biggest impact of turning 40 is mental. It forces us to take a long look at ourselves and ask, *Am I the person I always wanted to be? Have I accomplished everything I set out to do?*

Those can be complicated questions, to be sure. So here's a more straightforward one. Ask yourself: "Am I running out of time—or is this the best time?" Your answer reveals a lot about your mindset.

Why does your mindset matter? Because turning 40 hits us all differently. And before we talk about how to build physical strength, we need to talk about how to build mental strength. Having a positive outlook will help you face obstacles as you age and benefit your overall health. Research shows that, when compared with pessimists, optimists live 11 to 15 percent longer, sleep better, and are more likely to have better cardiovascular health.

Just like building muscle—that is, ripping apart muscle fibers, repairing them, and building them back stronger—constructing a truly strong mindset only comes after setbacks. And folks, I've had plenty of those.

There was a time when I straight lied to myself. I thought I had everything under control. I was working too much and sleeping too little. I had recently gotten divorced. There was child support, alimony, college tuition. I had rent payments due, in both San Diego and Los Angeles. My social life was practically nonexistent. But I was getting it done, and so I thought all was cool.

For years, I told myself that I was fine. But the cracks were starting to show, even if I was slow to notice them. I gained weight. I had a bout with shingles. I started having panic attacks when I got on airplanes—and I was a world traveler!

It wasn't until a good friend made me realize my actual problem—I sucked at dealing with stress—that I finally started cultivating a stronger and more resilient mindset.

THAT MINDSET helped when, in December 2020, I took a pretty bad spill on my mountain bike. I had just sped down a dirt trail and was steering around a fence (okay, I might have been going

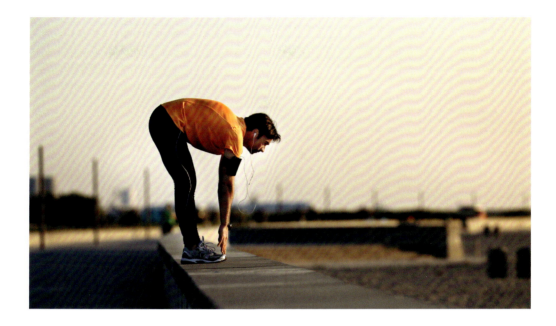

faster than I should have been) when suddenly my handlebars and pedal clipped the fence pole. The bike came to a halt, but I flew over my handlebars and landed on my chest. The backpack that I was wearing flew off my back and through the air. At first, I thought my gear had taken the worst of the fall (I broke my heart rate monitor and later found out that I'd jacked up my computer and a hard drive), so I got up and rode home.

Later, I realized my injuries were more extensive than I thought. Sure, I could still exercise (squats, deadlifts, plyometrics), but even nine months later, I still couldn't do the thing I loved most: sprint.

Despite my limitations, I focused on the activities I could enjoy and focused on my recovery plan. Yes, I was frustrated because I couldn't sprint—but I was never down or depressed.

Look, I know that my body doesn't make my mind strong. It's my mind that makes my body strong. And I know that mentality is what got me through that setback.

It's the same for everyone. If you want to exercise but can't work up the motivation , you need to work on your mental game. If you throw out your back lifting, you need to stay optimistic if you ever want to head back to the gym.

Maybe this sounds strange

coming from a fitness trainer, but it's the truth: the strongest part of your body isn't a muscle—it's your mind. But don't get it twisted. Some of you may see the word "mindset" or "mental approach" and instantly think "mental health."

Taking care of your mental health is a good thing. But that's not what I'm talking about here. I'm talking about the mentality and approach you need to take toward fitness as a man over 40. If you don't have a plan for how you're going to approach the next half of your life, you'll be in for some tough times. Throughout this book I'll give you the tools you need to tackle all of it with ease.

YOUR BODY AFTER 40

Let's talk about what 40 really is. Because we don't just turn 40 and then suddenly have a bunch of issues we didn't have yesterday. Let's break aging down into two categories: chronological age and biological age.

Our **chronological age** is the number of years, months, days, hours, and seconds that we've been alive. Unless we activate the flux capacitor on our DeLorean and get that 1.21 gigawatts, it's impossible to change our chronological age, no matter how active and healthy we are.

We can, however, slow down our **biological age**—the measurement of how much we've aged that's largely influenced by lifestyle habits. There's no simple formula that can calculate your biological age, but you can start by asking yourself a few questions: Do you exercise? Eat a healthy diet? Get enough sleep? If so, you might be biologically younger than someone who shares the same birthday with you, but doesn't have the same healthy lifestyle.

This book will help you turn back the clock on your biological age. Simply put, it's about getting older, but staying young.

If you want to avoid injury, supercharge your energy, and never slow down, you'll have to focus on more than just building muscle. Don't get me wrong—strength is important. But before you can properly build strength, you'll have to hone two things that you're probably overlooking: mobility and stability.

Here's why.

OUR FITNESS DECLINES WITH AGE

There's no getting around it: We will all lose some muscle as we get older. But not as much as you might think. Age-related muscle loss, known as sarcopenia, doesn't really begin for most people until about the age of 50. Even then, we only tend to lose about 1 percent of our muscle mass and 3 percent of our strength each year, according to a study by researchers at McMaster University.

In my opinion, the number one thing that's preventing men over the age of 40 from staying in shape is their lifestyle. Specifically, their sedentary lifestyle. I put a lot of the blame on computers and smartphones. Don't get me wrong: electronic media is great. But it's also given us the bent, kyphotic posture of a Neanderthal. It's as if we've evolved to walk upright only to descend back down into our hunched-over ancestors.

Of course, life gets in the way, too. When we were younger, we might have had more time to play sports or go to the gym. Now, all too many of us are juggling one (or two, or three) jobs and family responsibilities, as well as cooking, cleaning, and other tasks. But that doesn't mean that your health should come last on your list of priorities—something that I see all too often.

When your car makes a rattling noise, what do you do? Take it to a mechanic. When your sink springs a leak, what do you do? Call a plumber. Now—what do you do when you hurt your lower back? Most people I know either ignore the pain and work around it (trainers call this "compensating," by the way) or they stop exercising altogether.

I can't tell you how many times someone has called me and said they can't come in for a workout. They'll say, "Coach, I sprained my ankle. I can't exercise today." I tell them, "That's okay, today's an upper body day."

Folks, there's never a reason to stop exercising. And it's never too late to start. The more muscle you build now, the less you'll have to lose. The more you take care of your body today, the more energy you'll have tomorrow. The better shape you're in now, the healthier you'll be in the future.

In other words, you might be over 40, but if you take care of your body, you'll feel a hell of a lot younger. And isn't that the point, really?

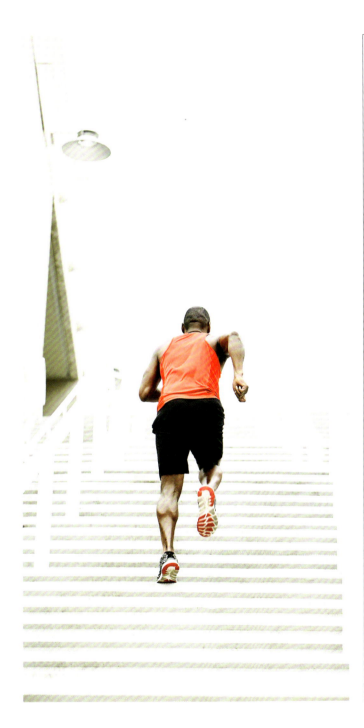

THE 2 TYPES OF MOVEMENTS EVERY GUY OVER 40 NEEDS

You might think the key to never slowing down is to maintain as much muscle as possible. But that power will fizzle if you're easily injured. Bulletproof your body by focusing on movements in two key categories: mobility and stability.

Mobility

Your body needs to move every day in order to keep working the right way. But over the course of four-plus decades, you've likely limited your daily movement to just a handful of positions. Ignoring all other potential ways your body can move leaves you susceptible to injury. That's where mobility exercises come in handy. Mobility is a joint's ability to move freely through its full range of motion without pain. Exercises like the Spiderman Lunge on page 54 or Superman Hold on page 80 can help you preserve ease of movement. They'll lubricate tight hips, relax your back, and stave off neck pains, too. Best of all, they don't take long to do.

Stability

Stability is your foundation. It's your ability to remain balanced. We all learned it as a kid, but it requires upkeep as we get older. Research shows that stability training can significantly reduce your risk of injury, plus it makes building strength a lot easier. The less stable you are, the less force you'll be able to produce. Stability moves, like the series of lunges you'll learn later on in this book, challenge your balance and help you remain anchored as you move through daily life. Work these into your regular routine and you'll be unshakeable.

MOVEMENT. MATTERS.

So where does that leave us? We have to make more time for movement. And specifically, we need to relearn how to move.

Movement is more vital to our health and well-being than any other factor besides good nutrition. Not just practicing but perfecting movement puts the life in living.

Does that sound fanatical? Well, call me converted. I am a faithful, devoted follower of what I like to call the First Church of Human Movement. Its Word is sound and powerful. Bending, extending, squatting, twisting, balancing—this, folks, is what will keep us healthy for the next 40 years.

I'm what many might stereotype as a "functional fitness" trainer. What I do, though, is all about performance, no matter the activity. I do whatever it takes to help athletes move and perform better. If that means Olympic lifts, I teach the clean-and-jerk and the snatch and all the exercises that go along with those. If that means sprinting, the athletes will find themselves repeating everything from figure-4 cycles to over-speed hurdle hops.

Folks, I've done plenty of "cave" work and participated in more than my share of National Bench and Triceps Days. All of that—the benching, squats, and deadlifts—are great. But there's

nothing I do or want to do that requires me to push weight up from my chest (there was actually a two-decade span, from 1999 to 2019, where I didn't bench press) or put ungodly amounts of stress on my back. I still deadlift (mostly with a trap bar) because that lift checks a lot of functional boxes. The older I've gotten, the smarter I've become about my training. You don't have to prove anything to the youngsters at the gym. You just need to be ready to play.

I'm training to kitesurf in Tarifa, hike Mount Kilimanjaro, and learn Bachata and Kizomba. After all, why would we train to be in the best possible shape if not to increase the joy in life?

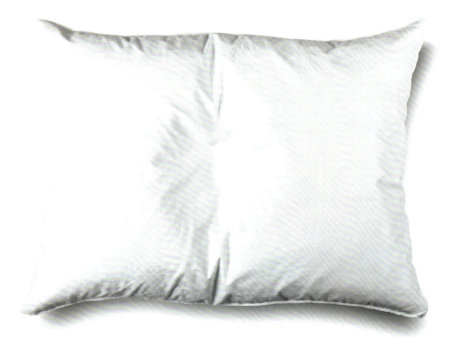

Start now, and here are all the benefits you can expect:

You'll Build Stronger Bones

As men get older, they also lose bone density, which can make them more susceptible to injuries and osteoporosis. And osteoporosis isn't just a "woman's problem"—about 10 to 25 percent of men are estimated to fracture a bone due to osteoporosis, according to a review in the journal *Bone Research*. This may be partly because men are living longer, say the researchers. Exercise, however, can help us maintain our bone health. One study by researchers from the University of Missouri found that doing resistance training for six months can increase bone density in men ages 25 to 60 years old.

You'll Reverse Brain Shrinkage

We may grow wiser with age, but our hippocampus—the area in the brain that helps with learning and memorization—grows smaller. Yes, another side effect of adding candles to our birthday cake. But what were we saying again? Oh, yes—luckily, exercise has the ability to reverse brain shrinkage. One study by researchers at the Salk Institute found that when people ages 55 to 80 participated in a year-long aerobic exercise program, they increased the volume in their hippocampus by 2 percent.

You'll Maintain More Muscle

There's no outrunning sarcopenia, the muscle loss that occurs as we age. For most of us, the biggest losses happen starting in our mid-60s, but it can also happen as early as our 40s.

Some of this is natural, and some of this is genetic, but another big culprit is inactivity. When it comes to movement, humans either use it or lose it. (More on that later.) When we stop doing certain movements—like pullups on the playground, for example—our brains stop firing the neurons that help us complete those movements. The result is that, over time, our bodies "forget" how to perform them.

The best way to attack sarcopenia is to move more. And not just more often—we need to literally move more, too. Lift something relatively heavy. Put it somewhere new. Move it again. And again. And again. In other words: Exercise.

You'll Burn More Calories

When we were young, we used to play pickup basketball games or ride our bikes—now, those things have fallen by the wayside. But when we don't work out, we lose muscle, and that, in turn, means we're likely burning less calories on a daily basis. Want to burn more calories at rest? Build more muscle.

You'll Sleep Better

Chances are, you're probably skimping on sleep. According to the latest statistics, about 35 to 40 percent of Americans ages 45 to 64 say they sleep fewer than 7 hours a night. Blame work stress, money stress, family stress, or any kind of stress. And then there are the physical culprits: arthritis, backaches, hip pain. The good news, though, is that exercise can improve sleep quality and shorten the amount of time it takes you to fall asleep, according to a 2017 research review.

You'll Preserve More Testosterone

After their 30th birthday, men tend to lose testosterone at a rate of 1 percent each year. That means that by the time we're 40, our bodies may be producing about 10 percent less testosterone than they did when we were 25. Still, some research suggests that this decline in T isn't solely a result of our chronological age. Rather, some of it is due to our biological age—our cumulative levels of stress, injuries, health conditions, and more. Want

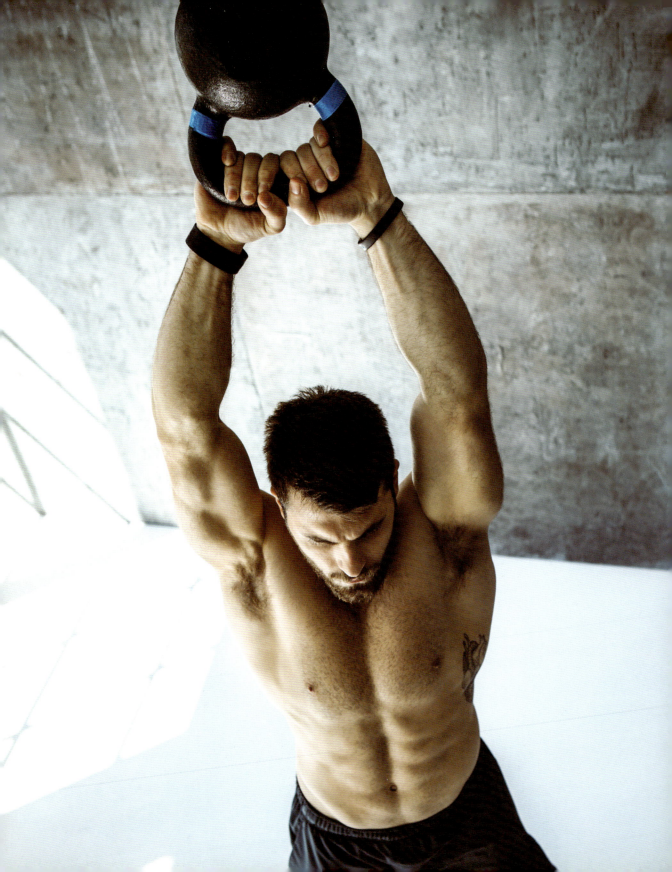

to increase your testosterone? Grab a heavy weight and start lifting it.

You'll Have Better Sex

Sexual dysfunction doesn't necessarily happen because of age—conditions like stress can also play a role. Exercise, however, can help ease stress and boost performance. A study in *The Journal of Sexual Medicine* found that exercise is linked to better erectile and sexual function.

You'll Feel Better Mentally, Too

I could cite studies about the mood-boosting benefits of exercise. But let's be honest—once we turn 40, it's probably going to take more than a few workouts a week to keep our mental health in the best possible shape. Once I turned 40, I became very conscious of the fact that, most likely, more of my life was behind me than in front of me.

My advice: Don't run from it. I've seen that strategy lead to midlife crises. I've seen divorces (and experienced one as well). I've seen nervous breakdowns. I've seen men isolate themselves from the world. I'm also a life coach as well as a fitness coach, so I have a clear understanding of the power that our mind has over us. Accepting the aging process can be very therapeutic. But what helps us live an amazingly full life is the planning we do to make that life possible.

Of course, I also believe that heavy lifting can be a big part of that therapy. Take your stress out on the weights, not on the world around you.

BONUS: You Might Boost Your Immune System

Our immune systems decline when our bodies fail to produce as many infection-fighting cells as it did when we were younger. But staying active as you get older may help slow the age-related decline to our immune health, according to a 2018 study. The researchers also concluded that regular exercise may also reduce your chances of being sickened with a bacterial or viral infection.

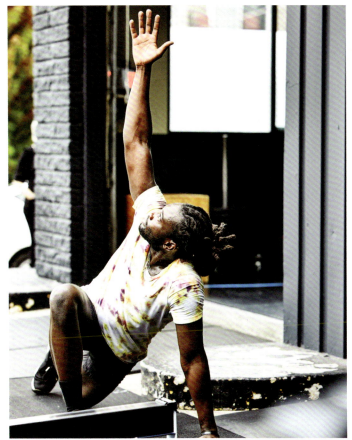

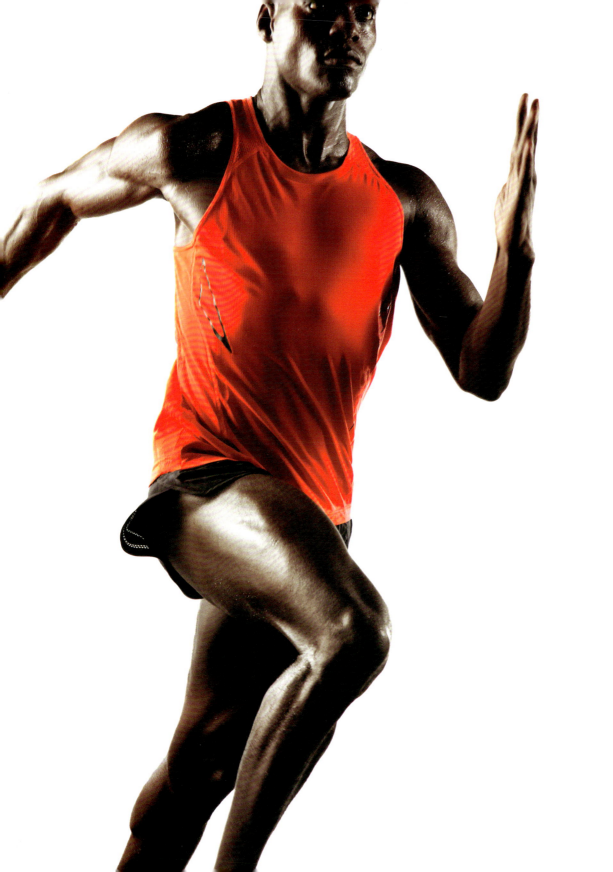

CHAPTER

02

IN THIS CHAPTER, YOU'LL...

MASTER YOUR BODY'S BASIC MOVEMENTS

UNCOVER (AND REPAIR) YOUR BODY'S STRUCTURAL WEAKNESSES

BULLETPROOF YOURSELF AGAINST INJURY

FIND YOUR
STARTING POINT

AS I PREVIOUSLY mentioned, your chronological age and biological age are two different things. Your body may technically be 40, but that doesn't mean it functions the same as every other 40-year-old's. That's where finding your baseline makes all the difference. Identifying your unique fitness starting point sets you up for success on your quest to defy your chronological age and become truly unstoppable. With a few simple assessments, you will better equip your body and mind for whatever obstacles arise.

The tests in this chapter will, first and foremost, help you establish a strong mindset, a critical component for any fitness endeavor. They will help you manage your expectations of what you can and can't yet do. Why is this so crucial to staying motivated? Knowing your existing limits means you won't be blindsided by setbacks. You won't sign up for a 10K only to quit halfway

through training because you can't run like you used to. Defeat can be demotivating. So don't put yourself in a position to be defeated. Establish your physical limits first, then work to gradually redefine them.

In addition to helping you avoid a bruised ego, these assessments will also help you avoid an aching back (and knee, and shoulder, and everything else). Each exercise and the questions that follow it are designed to highlight deficiencies. Many of the movements are isolated, dialed-back versions of moves you might make while playing a sport or training in the gym. They allow you to test your capabilities without exposing yourself to injury.

Your findings will evolve into a roadmap for long-term fitness success: You'll know exactly what you need to work on most, and exactly what you should avoid until you've passed each test. Let's say, for example, that you struggle with the shoulder

mobility test on page 27. Now you know you should skip the windup pitch next time you're playing catch with the kids.

In the ideal world, you'd head to a trainer to have these assessments done. But if you take your time and work through this chapter and pay extra-close attention to the way you move, you'll have a strong idea of where you are. The tests in this chapter are the same ones I've used to assess many clients over the years, and I learned them from a variety of sources. Some are pulled from the Selective Functional Movement Assessment (SFMA), designed by Gray Cook and a few other insanely smart movement specialists. The rest are derived from the movement patterns that everyone does during their daily lives.

Together, they'll help you identify the movement inefficiencies that are holding you back from being your most unstoppable self.

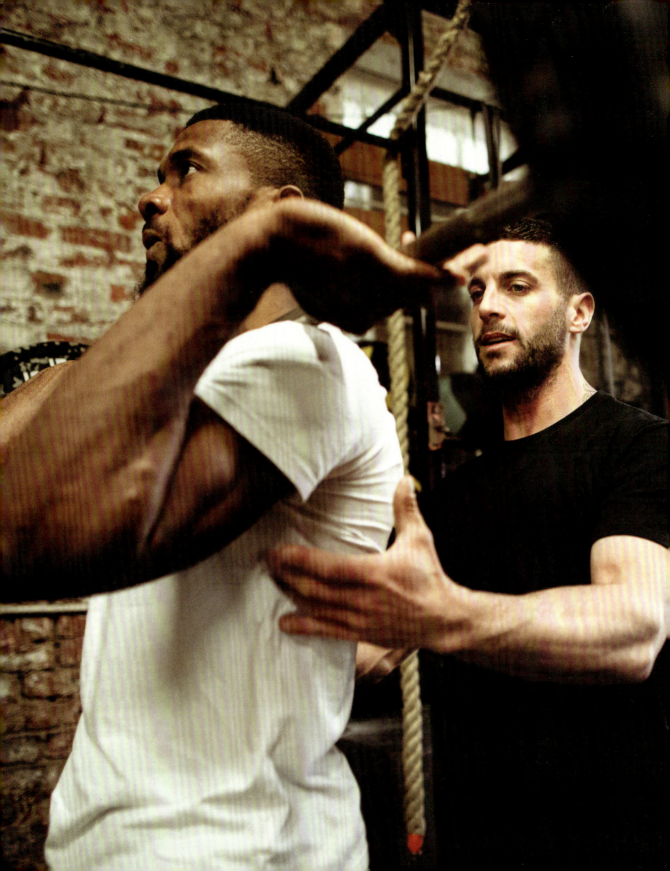

14 EXERCISES TO FIND
YOUR STARTING POINT

TAKE THE FOLLOWING TESTS, THEN ASK YOURSELF THE "WHAT TO LOOK FOR" QUESTIONS. IF YOU ANSWER "YES" TO ANY, TRY THE "IMPROVE IT" TIPS AND REPEAT THE TEST WEEKLY UNTIL YOU PERFORM IT SUCCESSFULLY.

BREATHING

WHAT IT TESTS: How well you breathe while you're relaxed.

TAKE THE TEST: Lie on your back with your knees bent and feet flat. Breathe for 20 to 30 seconds to get relaxed. Then ask someone to observe you for 1 minute.

WHAT TO LOOK FOR:
▶ Did your belly inflate before your abdomen?
▶ Did your ribcage or abdomen inflate second?
▶ Was your chest the last area to rise?
▶ Did you take more than 16 breaths during the minute?

IMPROVE IT:
01. If your abdomen fails to inflate first, lie on your back with your knees bent and feet flat. Put a hand on your chest and a hand on your stomach. Breathe in through your nose, concentrating on making the hand on your abdomen rise while the other remains stationary.

02. If your abdomen still fails to inflate first, lie on your back with your knees bent at 90 degrees and feet against a wall or on a chair. Pull your shoulders down and press your lower back into the ground. Place your hands on your stomach and chest again. Breathe in through your nose, again trying to raise the hand on your abdomen while keeping the other hand stationary.

Rolling Patterns

This series of 4 movements helps you assess your level of core stability. They can all be improved with one simple exercise, which you'll find on the next page.

UPPER BODY SUPINE-TO-PRONE

WHAT IT TESTS: Your core's ability to be simultaneously dynamic and stable while you rotate your body from back to stomach, moving from your outstretched hands down to your feet.

TAKE THE TEST: Lie on your back with your arms overhead and feet hip-width apart. Imagine that your body is dead from your waist through your feet—any lower body movement should only happen as a consequence of the upper body moving. To start the movement, raise your head and rotate it to the left as if you're smelling your left armpit. Starting with your right arm, reach to the left, followed by your head, then your neck, then your right shoulder, then your chest, until you're on your stomach. Return to the starting position and perform the rolling pattern to the right.

WHAT TO LOOK FOR:
▶ Did you use a jerking motion to start the movement?
▶ Did you get stuck?
▶ Did you use a jerking motion to urge your midsection to roll?
▶ Did you use your glutes, knees, or feet to help you roll?

UPPER BODY PRONE-TO-SUPINE

WHAT IT TESTS: Your core's ability to be simultaneously dynamic and stable while you rotate your body from stomach to back, moving from your outstretched hands down to your feet.

TAKE THE TEST: Lie on your stomach with your left arm overhead and your right arm out to the side. Your feet should be hip-width apart. Think of your body as dead from your waist through your feet—any lower body movement should only happen as a consequence of the upper body moving. In rolling to the left, turn your head to your right, looking at your right hand. Then raise your right hand and arm so that they extend up and over your back toward your left side. Keep your eyes on your right hand and follow it with your head as it continues to the ground. Your lower body should stay relaxed until the rotation of your upper body begins pulling your lower over as well. Return to the starting position and perform the rolling pattern to the right.

WHAT TO LOOK FOR:
▶ Did you use a jerking motion to start the movement?
▶ Did you get stuck?
▶ Did you use a jerking motion to urge the midsection to roll?
▶ Did you use your glutes, knees, or feet to help you roll?

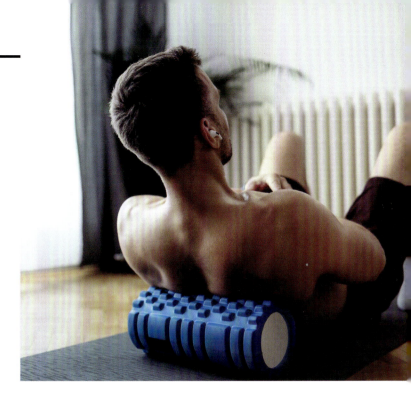

LOWER BODY SUPINE-TO-PRONE

WHAT IT TESTS: Your core's ability to be simultaneously dynamic and stable while you rotate your body from your back to your stomach, moving from the bottoms of your heels up to the tips of your out-stretched hands.

TAKE THE TEST: Lie on your back with your arms overhead and feet hip-width apart. Think of your body as dead from the waist through the hands—any upper body movement should only happen as a conse-quence of the lower body moving. Raise your right leg vertically and, keeping your left leg stationary, rotate it so your toes point left. Reach the right leg to the left until your hips begin rotating. As your hips rotate, your upper body will follow suit until your whole body is in a supine position. Repeat this while rolling to the right.

WHAT TO LOOK FOR:
▶ Did you use a jerking motion to start the movement?
▶ Did you get stuck?

LOWER BODY PRONE-TO-SUPINE

WHAT IT TESTS: Your core's ability to be simultaneously dynamic and stable while you rotate your body from your stomach to your back, moving from the bottoms of your heels up to the tips of your outstretched hands.

TAKE THE TEST: Lie on your stomach with your arms overhead and feet hip-width apart. Think of your body as dead from your waist through your feet—any lower body movement should only happen as a conse-quence of the upper body moving. In rolling to the left, raise your right leg in a diagonal over your left leg while keeping the left leg stationary. As your right leg reaches across your body, your hips should begin rotat-ing. As your hips rotate, your upper body will follow suit until your whole body is in a supine position. Repeat this while rolling to the right.

WHAT TO LOOK FOR:
▶ Did you use a jerking motion to start the movement?
▶ Did you get stuck?
▶ Did you use a jerking motion to get your midsection to roll?
▶ Did you use any part of your shoulders, elbows or hands to help you roll?

IMPROVE IT:
01. This movement can help improve each of the upper and lower body rolling patterns. If these pat-terns are challenging, get a half foam roller or a rolled-up towel, and place it under your back or chest, parallel to your spine, on the same side as the limb you begin the movement with. It should go under your back for the back-to-stomach pattern and under your chest for the stomach-to-back pattern. Your torso will be at an angle during the starting position—this will shorten the distance you have to roll and make the exercise easier to do. Perform the rolling pattern using the same movements as before. Decrease the angle if it's too easy. Increase it if it is too difficult.

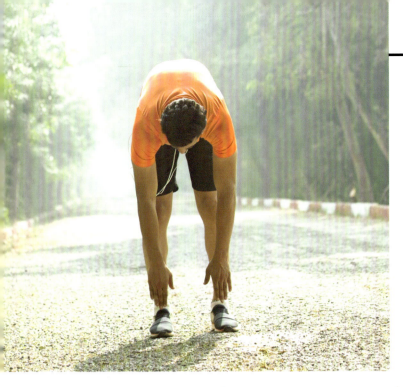

TOE TOUCH

WHAT IT TESTS: If you have a good range of motion in your hips, glutes, hamstrings, and spine.

TAKE THE TEST: Bend forward at your hips and try to touch your toes without flexing your knees.

WHAT TO LOOK FOR:
► When you were as bent over as you could get, were your hands still above your feet?
► When you were bent over, did your hips stick out behind you instead of staying above your feet?
► Did your spine curve more in one section of your back, instead of creating an even arc?
► Did your legs bend, even a little?

IMPROVE IT:
01. Lie on your back with your legs straight. Raise your right leg as high as you can. Have a friend take note of how high you can lift your leg. Repeat with your left leg. If both of your legs reached the same height, move to the next step. If your legs reached drastically different heights, you have an asymmetry (for example, you may have muscle imbalances or weaknesses, motor control issues, or joint dysfunctions), and may need to consult a physical therapist or other movement specialist to be certain.

02. Grab a couple of bath towels and a yoga block. (If you don't have a yoga block, another bath towel will work.) Place the rolled towel on the ground and stand on it so that your heels are elevated and your toes are down. Take the yoga block or roll up a second towel and place it between your thighs. Squeeze the block or towel between your thighs and keep squeezing it throughout the movements of hinging your hips to bend over and touch your toes. If you have to flex your knees to touch, do so. As you return to the standing position, reach with your hands high above your head while continuing to squeeze the block or towel. That's 1 rep. Do 5 reps with your heels up and your toes on the ground, followed by 5 reps with your toes elevated and your heels on the ground.

BACK BEND

WHAT IT TESTS: If you have good range of motion in your shoulders, hips, and spine.

TAKE THE TEST: Stand tall with your arms above your head. Bend as far backward as possible while keeping your feet planted firmly on the ground.

WHAT TO LOOK FOR:
► Did your upper arms shift so that they were in front of or behind your ears?
► Did your hip bones (a.k.a. ASIS, the bones at the top front of your pelvis) move in front of your toes?
► Did your shoulders extend back past your heels?
► Was the curve in your spine uneven?

IMPROVE IT:
01. Do the Spiderman Lunge with Rotation (page 55).

02. Lie on your back and place the foam roller horizontally under your shoulder blades. Support your neck and head by clasping your hands behind your head. Flare your elbows out to the side, supporting your head and neck. Do not fold your elbows in front of your head. Keep your head and neck in line with your spine and your butt on the ground. Think of the spine in terms of individual sections. Roll back to each section five times. Keep repeating this rolling pattern until you reach the bottom of your rib cage.

TOTAL-BODY ROTATION RIGHT & LEFT

WHAT IT TESTS: That you have a good range of motion in your neck, thoracic spine, hips, pelvis, knees, and feet.

TAKE THE TEST: Stand tall with your feet together, toes forward, and your arms hanging by your sides. Turn your body as far to the right as possible, while keeping your feet in place. Check your posture. Then repeat this movement while turning your body to the left.

WHAT TO LOOK FOR:
▶ Do your feet shift position or move?
▶ Was there any loss of height? (For example, your trunk flexed.)
▶ When you rotated left, could you see your right shoulder? When you rotated right, could you see your left shoulder?
▶ Could you rotate less than 50 degrees in your shoulders and in your torso?

IMPROVE IT:
01. Do the Spiderman Lunge with Rotation (page 55).

02. Do the Carioca exercise (page 59).

SINGLE-LEG STANCE RIGHT & LEFT

WHAT IT TESTS: Your ability to stabilize one side while retaining awareness of your body's relationship to the space around it. When you close your eyes, this assessment tests your balance, spatial awareness, and ability to understand the directions your body is moving.

TAKE THE TEST: Stand tall with your feet together. Lift your right leg so that your thigh is at least parallel to the ground and your knee is bent at a 90-degree angle. Hold that position for 10 seconds. Then close your eyes and hold that position for 10 seconds. Repeat both positions with your left leg.

WHAT TO LOOK FOR:
▶ Did your support foot (the one on the ground) change position?
▶ Was there a loss of height?
▶ Did you lose your posture?
▶ Did your arms flail?
▶ Could you hold the position for less than 10 seconds, eyes open and closed?

IMPROVE IT:
01. Stand upright and flex your right glute while simultaneously flexing your abdominal core muscles. Raise your left foot off the ground while maintaining the flex in both the glute and core. Remember your breathing—in through the nose, feeling your abdomen expand (yes, even when you're bracing your core muscles).

NOTE: Think of your body as a chessboard: The glutes are the kings of stability, and the core is the queen. The chess match is over when the king gets caught—which makes the king the most important piece on the board. But the queen is the most versatile piece on the board. When it comes to balance before we make a move, the brain tells the core—the queen—to shift the body's center of gravity. Once that center of gravity has been shifted, the brain tells the glutes to take over and provide stability. Once that happens, the core is able to help the body maintain its center of gravity during other movements. Working together, they help us maintain stability in most situations whether our eyes are open or closed.

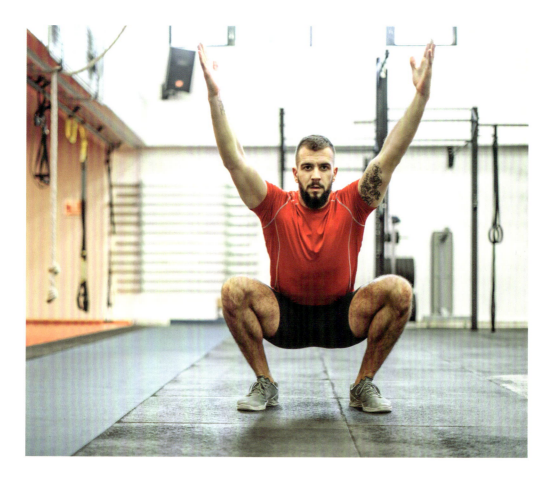

OVERHEAD DEEP SQUAT

WHAT IT TESTS: Your hip, knee, ankle, shoulder, and thoracic spine mobility.

THE TEST: Stand tall with your feet shoulder-width apart. Raise your arms above your head with your elbows extended. Then allow your hips and knees to flex, and let your body descend to its deepest position.

WHAT TO LOOK FOR:
▶ Did your heels come off the ground?
▶ Did your knees face a different direction than your toes?
▶ Do your knees travel past your feet?
▶ Were your thighs higher than parallel with the ground?

IMPROVE IT:

01. Sit on the edge of a chair with your feet flat on the ground, shoulder-width apart. Keeping your core braced, lean your torso slightly forward and push through your heels to stand up. Over time, lean forward less and start on a lower surface (such as a heavy box).

02. Hold a dumbbell, kettlebell, or heavy backpack in front of you at shoulder level while standing tall with your feet shoulder-width apart. Hinge your hips and descend into a squat position. The weight will counteract your movement and balance your center of gravity as you descend. Doing this often allows you to descend lower. As you get stronger, use a lighter weight.

SHOULDER MOBILITY

WHAT IT TESTS: The mobility in your upper extremities (shoulders, arms, wrists) as well as the extension in your thoracic spine.

TAKE THE TEST: Stand tall with your feet together, hands near your sides. In one fluid motion, take your left hand and reach up your back to touch the bottom of the right shoulder blade. Then take your left hand and reach up, then down to touch the top of your right shoulder blade. Then do the same movements with the right hand.

WHAT TO LOOK FOR:
▶ Did your right hand stop before reaching the top or bottom of your left shoulder blade?
▶ Did your left hand stop before reaching the top or bottom of your right shoulder blade?
▶ Do you have to wiggle or crawl your right hand into position?
▶ Do you have to wiggle or crawl your left hand into position?

IMPROVE IT:
01. Use a foam roller to roll your upper back. Lie on your back and place the foam roller horizontally under your shoulder blades. Support your neck and head by clasping your hands behind your head. Flare your elbows out to the side, supporting your head and neck. Do not fold your elbows in front of your head. Keep your head and neck in line with your spine and your butt on the ground. Think of the spine in terms of individual sections. Roll back to each section five times. Keep repeating this rolling until you reach the bottom of your rib cage. This can be intensified by stretching your arms over your head, in line with your spine, and repeating the movements.

02. Use a foam roller to roll the lats and shoulders. Lie on your right side and place the foam roller horizontally under your upper right lat. Stretch your right arm above your head so that the arm is in line with the spine and torso. Gently roll your body up and down the length of the lat while rotating back and forth to hit the lat from multiple angles.

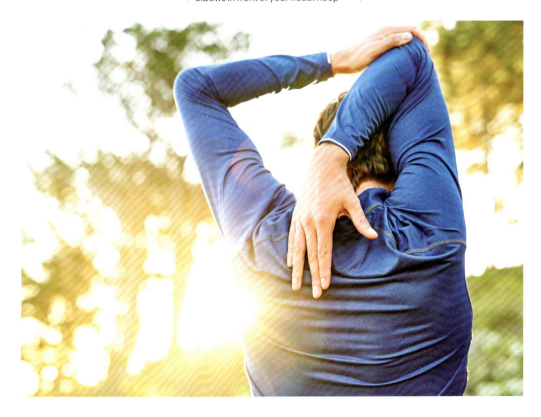

SKIPPING FORWARD & BACKWARD

WHAT IT TESTS: A higher-level cross-crawling pattern.

TAKE THE TEST: Skip forward for 10 yards, then skip backward for 10 yards.

WHAT TO LOOK FOR:
▶ Did your right hand and left knee lose synchronicity with each other?
▶ Did your left hand and right foot lose synchronicity?
▶ Did you sway or lean to one side?
▶ Were your arms loose or bent?
▶ Was there a step-hop, step-hop rhythm, with no disjointed or choppy skips?

IMPROVE IT:
01. Skipping has a repeated step-hop motion. Instead of simply stepping and hopping, take a step forward with your left foot, and then as your right leg comes forward, raise your right knee, hop off your left foot and tap the inside of your right knee with your left hand. As your right foot touches the ground and your left leg comes forward, hop off your right leg and tap the inside of your left knee with your right hand. Keep repeating that motion moving forward. Do the same knee tapping while skipping backward.

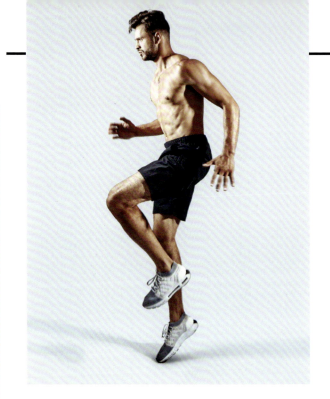

SINGLE-LEG HOPPING LEFT & RIGHT

WHAT IT TESTS: Your total-body coordination, in a dynamic fashion, while on one foot.

TAKE THE TEST: Hop on one foot for 10 yards, then turn around and hop back on the other foot to the starting point.

WHAT TO LOOK FOR:
▶ Did your right hand and left knee move forward in synch with each other?
▶ Did your left hand lose synchronicity with your right knee as it moved forward?
▶ Did your arms hang straight by your sides instead of moving simultaneously as if you were rowing?
▶ Did either of your feet land anywhere but the ball of your foot on any of the hops?
▶ Did the swing of your free leg fall out of unison with your torso's movement?
▶ Did your torso tend to lean forward or backward?

IMPROVE IT:
01. Stand tall on your right leg with your left leg bent at the knee. Swing your left leg back and forth while maintaining the bend in your knee. Your left knee should travel in front and behind your body's center of mass BUT your left foot should never extend in front of the left knee. Make sure the right arm moves in sync with the left leg. Do this for 10 reps. Repeat this motion with the right leg.

02. Stand tall on your right leg with your left leg bent at the knee. Start with your left foot behind the body. Swing the left leg forward, while maintaining the flexed knee. As your left knee comes forward, hop on your right leg. Your left knee and right arm must move forward and return to the starting position in the same amount of time it takes your right leg to hop once. Do this for 10 reps. Repeat with the right leg swinging.

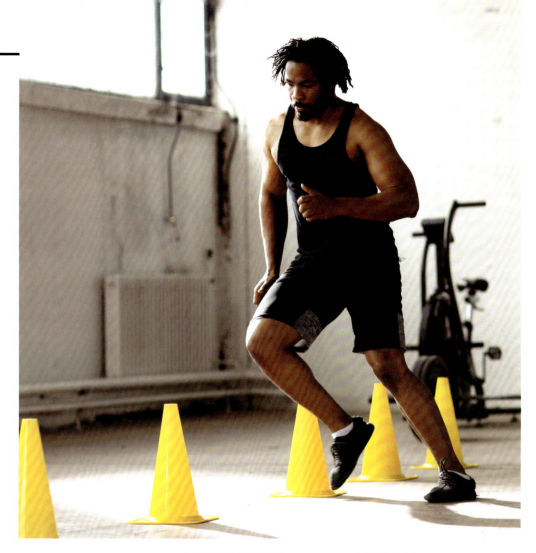

SHUFFLING RIGHT & LEFT

WHAT IT TESTS: Your ability to efficiently shift your bodyweight while moving in a side-to-side motion.

TAKE THE TEST: Face a direction perpendicular to your direction of travel. Shuffle 10 yards. Then shuffle the 10 yards back while facing the same direction.

WHAT TO LOOK FOR:
▶ Did your feet lose their perpendicular position to the direction you were traveling at any point?
▶ Do you move into a squat or do your hands come to your sides? (This isn't a typical basketball drill.)
▶ Did your face turn away from the direction perpendicular to the one you were moving in?
▶ Did the front of your torso point in any direction except perpendicular to the direction your body was moving?
▶ Did the coordination of your arms and feet break down?
▶ Do your feet touch in the middle?
▶ Did your feet slide instead of hop?

IMPROVE IT:
01. Shuffle across the 10 yards without swinging your arms. Feel the gravity of the shoulders moving up and down. That will be your natural rhythm. Repeat the shuffling motion while letting your arms gently swing with the natural rhythm that you felt during the previous shuffle.

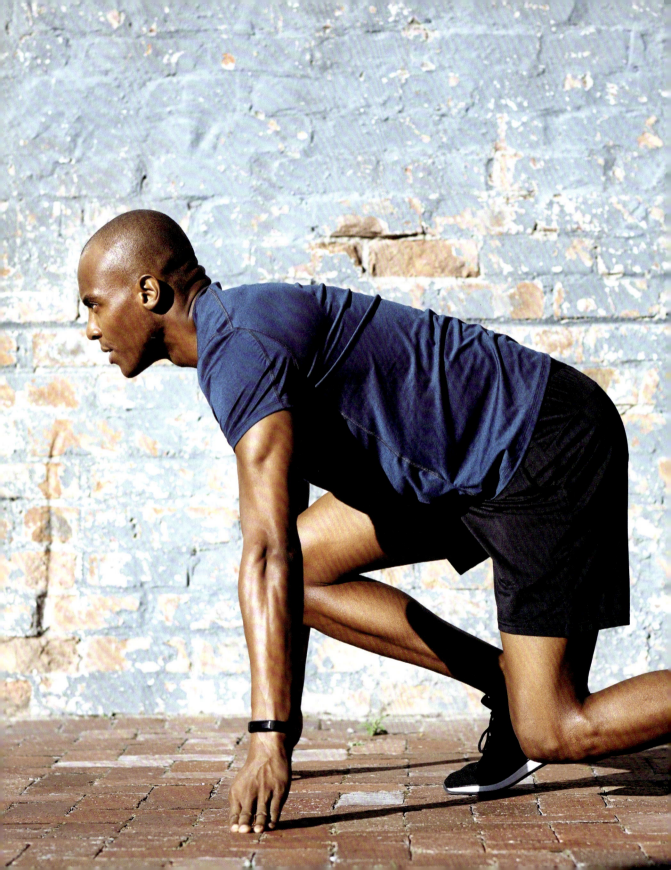

CHAPTER

03

BOOST YOUR WORKOUT RECOVERY

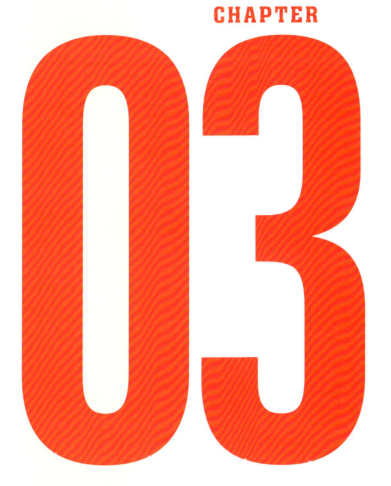

IN THIS CHAPTER, YOU'LL...

RECOVER FASTER FROM WORKOUTS (WITHOUT EXPENSIVE TOOLS)

PINPOINT EXACTLY WHAT YOU NEED TO EAT TO BOUNCE BACK FULLY

IMPROVE YOUR SLEEP HABITS AND DRIFT OFF FASTER

I'LL LET you in on a little secret I learned about recovery. There are two near-magical things you can do to bounce back after a workout.

The first thing? Get enough sleep.

GET SERIOUS ABOUT SLEEP

Every part of your body will benefit from a good night's sleep. Too little sleep can increase our blood pressure and stress levels, suppress our growth hormones, strain our heart health, and make it harder to focus and problem-solve. Even our mood and our attitude to others is compromised by a lack of shut-eye.

I've always known this—and yet, there was a time when I wasn't getting nearly enough sleep. In 2018, I was training for a photo shoot, trying to get in the best possible shape I could. But I was only averaging about 4 hours of sleep. And that was on a good night. I was groggy and sluggish. I was dragging by noon. I was hiding my yawns behind my hands while I trained people at the gym.

I did everything I could to sneak in a few more hours of sleep. I hit the snooze button. I tried meditation. Deep breathing. I took GABA, melatonin, magnesium, ZMA packs. Nothing worked. Finally, I tried a combination of THC and CBD gummies (I live in SoCal, folks. It's legal.) The first day I ate 5 milligrams of each and slept a whopping 8 hours.

Oh. My. Goodness.

Keep in mind that I have never taken a puff on a cigarette, much less gone near marijuana. But I was desperate, so I kept doing it. It worked, too, for a while. Then one day I went to the dispensary and found that the brand I was using had changed their formula. "New and improved," so to speak. Cool, I thought. Nothing wrong with improvement!

I got headaches for the next four nights. I went back to the store, looking for my old formula, only to find that they were no longer making it. I tried other brands, too. All of them gave me headaches.

So there I was, back to square one, averaging about 4 hours of sleep a night.

This continued until, one day, I confided in fellow trainer and hormone expert Janet Alexander that I had barely slept the night before. I just didn't get it, I said. I should have been exhausted—I spent the day training, did a leg workout at my gym, The Playground, and played Hooverball on the beach.

She asked me what I had eaten the night before. I told her I'd eaten a sizable salad and a lot of salmon.

"That's it?" she asked.

"Well, it was a lot of salad and salmon," I told her.

"After all that, you fed your body with rabbit food?" she asked. "Milo, Milo, Milo. Your body is freaking hungry! It's waking up at 2 a.m. saying, 'FEED ME.' You need to eat something substantial closer to bedtime."

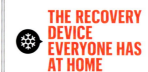

THE RECOVERY DEVICE EVERYONE HAS AT HOME

IF YOU'VE NEVER TRIED taking a contrast shower, let me tell you: It is the real deal. The next time you take a shower, turn the water to as cold as you can stand it and let the stream hit your muscles for about a minute (rotate your body a few times). Then, turn the water to warm (not crazy hot) and do the same thing for another minute. Keep switching the water from cold to hot, hot to cold for 8 to 10 minutes. Alternating between hot and cold water improves blood circulation (the heat moves your blood toward the skin, and the cold moves the blood away from the skin), and improved blood circulation can help fuel muscle growth. Plus, it also helps flush toxins from the body, including those from exercise.

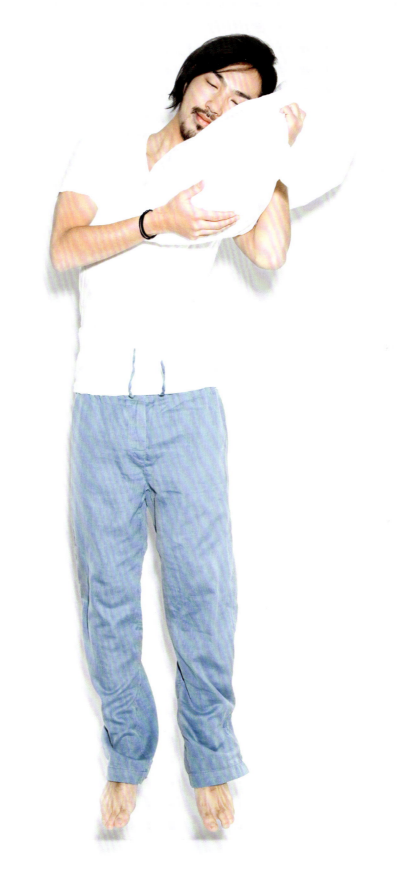

I ate a heaping plate of beef and veggies an hour before going to bed the next night. I slept eight hours.

You've probably already figured out that you can lift more and exercise longer when you get a good night's sleep. But folks, at this stage in our life, the consequences of too little sleep go way beyond a lack of gains in the gym. A 2012 review by German researchers found that our sleep-wake cycles play an important role in helping to produce key proteins that boost our immune system response—and that long-term sleep deprivation can increase inflammation.

Over time, too little sleep can also increase the risk of heart disease (the leading cause of death for men and women in the US), as well as diabetes, heart failure, heart attacks, and stroke. It can also interfere with your attention span, memory, and even sex drive, as well as contribute to depression.

Listen—we're not young anymore. We don't have the luxury of quickly bouncing back from an all-nighter. If we want to function at our best, we need to give our body and our mind every chance to do so. That doesn't mean getting precisely eight hours of sleep every night. It is going to vary for each of us—and it can vary from day to day depending on your exercise sessions, stress levels, and more.

Here's another way to look at it: Sleep deprivation has been used as a form of interrogation and torture. Why do that to yourself? If you have trouble dozing off, try these tips to fall asleep faster and stay asleep longer.

Change Your Lighting

From the lamps in your bedroom to the glow of your electronic devices, lighting affects

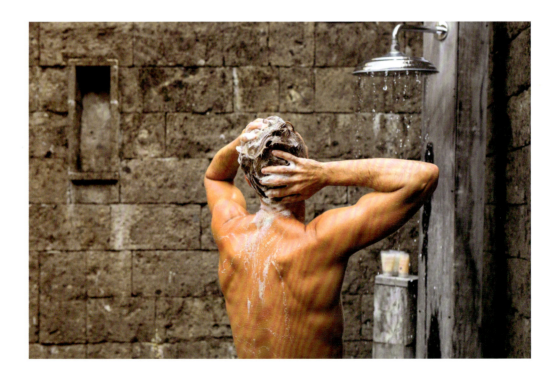

your ability to sleep. The melatonin hormone helps regulate your sleep-wake cycle and your exposure to light controls those hormone levels. When it's time to hit the hay, darkness is key. It might seem like the light from your phone or TV isn't messing with your ability to catch some rest, but it is. You should avoid looking at any bright screens up to two hours before you're hoping to fall asleep. It might be worth considering switching out your light bulbs. Smart bulbs like the Philips Hue line take these factors into account and can be customized to your needs so they won't affect your ability to fall asleep or fall back asleep if you happen to wake up in the middle of the night. If you need to turn on a light in the middle of the night, dimmer is better.

Shower At Night
You might want to rethink your daily routine if you're a morning shower person. There's evidence that cleaning yourself off at the end of the day can actually help you sleep better. The key is to time it correctly. Showering immediately before bed is actually not a good thing because the hot water raises your body temperature. Allowing your body to cool down before tucking yourself in for the night is the best way to do it. So grab your go-to soap of choice and hit

the shower if you're looking to get a good night's rest.

Practice Guided Meditation
Stressed out about your inability to sleep? Meditation has been shown to reduce cortisol levels, helping you feel less anxious and more relaxed—and thus, more likely to fall asleep. A 2015 study in *JAMA* found that mindfulness meditation helped improve sleep quality in older adults by reducing "worry, rumination, and mood disturbances." Try an app or other meditation product to help you get started.

Make Your Bed A Place For Sleep
If you've ever found yourself laying in bed unable to sleep, you've experience what researchers call "conditioned arousal," which is caused by doing things in bed that have trained your brain to keep you awake rather than fall asleep— like checking work email on your phone. So keep your bed a sleeping-only zone.

Crank Up The Air Conditioning
Studies have shown that sleeping in cooler temps is best for sleep. For optimal benefits, set your thermostat between 60 and 68 degrees Fahrenheit. This helps decrease your body's core

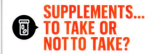

SUPPLEMENTS... TO TAKE OR NOT TO TAKE?

I'M NOT ANTI-SUPPLEMENT, but I'm pretty close to it. Truth be told, you can find most of the "supplements" you need in real foods. Instead of raiding GNC once a month, work on keeping several nutritious foods in your regular diet rotation. Chicken breast and quinoa cover your protein and fiber. Kiwi, a terrifically underrated superfood, delivers vitamin C and plenty of antioxidants, and a beet and arugula salad can deliver the nitrates you need for exercise performance and heart health. Try integrating each of these into your diet at least once a week. It beats relying on shakes for your nutrition . . . although that doesn't mean you should never touch a supplement. It doesn't hurt to keep a few protein bars in your gym bag at all times. They're a perfect bailout (and much better than a candy bar) when you're on the go and short on time.

temperature, triggering a process that initiates sleep.

Have A Consistent Schedule
Sleeping in on the weekend feels pretty great, but the habit may explain why you have a hard

time falling asleep. The National Sleep Foundation recommends going to bed and waking up at the same time every day—yes, weekends too! This helps keep your body's internal clock regular, which makes it easier to fall—and stay—asleep.

REFUEL STRATEGICALLY

Now for the second near-magical thing you can do to bounce back after a workout: Eat well.

I thought I was eating the right things. And for the most part, I was. But I wasn't eating the right things at the right times. As it turns out, I had to go back to the science.

Now, I am not a nutritionist. I do, however, have good friends who are nutritionists. They've helped me figure out how many calories I need to eat, and when I need to eat them. Short of seeing a nutritionist—and if you can, I highly recommend it—you can also use some simple calculations to get a good ballpark number for yourself.

The first thing you'll need to do is calculate your basal

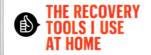

THE RECOVERY TOOLS I USE AT HOME

I HAVE PLENTY OF RECOVERY tools at home that I use. For each one, I could point you to an expert who swears by them, but I could also point you to an expert who chalks up any benefits to placebo effect. My advice: If it feels good and seems to help, use it. Here are the therapeutic devices I use:

- Foam rollers
- Hypervolt massage guns
- Compex electronic stimulation units
- The Stick therapeutic body massager

metabolic rate (BMR), or resting metabolic rate—the amount of energy you'll use if you do nothing but sit in bed all day. One equation you can use is the Harris-Benedict Equation (below).

For me, that came out to: 66 + (6.23 x 220 lb.) + (12.7 x 72 in.) – (6.8 x 47) = 2,031.4 calories a day. Translation: I burn a little

over 2,000 calories a day doing absolutely nothing.

But because none of us spends every waking minute of the day in bed, we have to go one step further and calculate our daily activity expenditure. We can do this by multiplying our BMR by one of the following numbers:

- ► Little to no exercise: **1.2**
- ► 1 to 3 days per week of moderate-intensity exercise: **1.555**
- ► Four days a week of moderate- to high-intensity exercise: **1.725**
- ► More than four days of high-intensity exercise each week: **1.9**

For me, that's 2,031.4 x 1.725 = 3,504.17 calories.

Finally, if you want to be as accurate as possible, you can multiply your BMR by 10 percent for the thermal effect of food (TEF), or the amount of calories that our body uses simply to metabolize the food we eat, and add that number to your energy expenditure. For me, that's 2,031.4 x 0.10 = 203.1.

Add it all together, and my total daily energy expenditure is 3,707.8 calories a day.

Now, I believe it's important for every athlete to know how many calories they need. But when you're 40 or older, your metabolism slows down, and you can't get away with eating anything you want anymore.

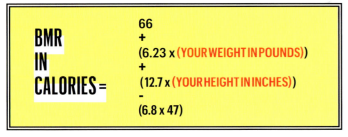

BMR IN CALORIES =

66
+
(6.23 x (YOUR WEIGHT IN POUNDS))
+
(12.7 x (YOUR HEIGHT IN INCHES))
–
(6.8 x 47)

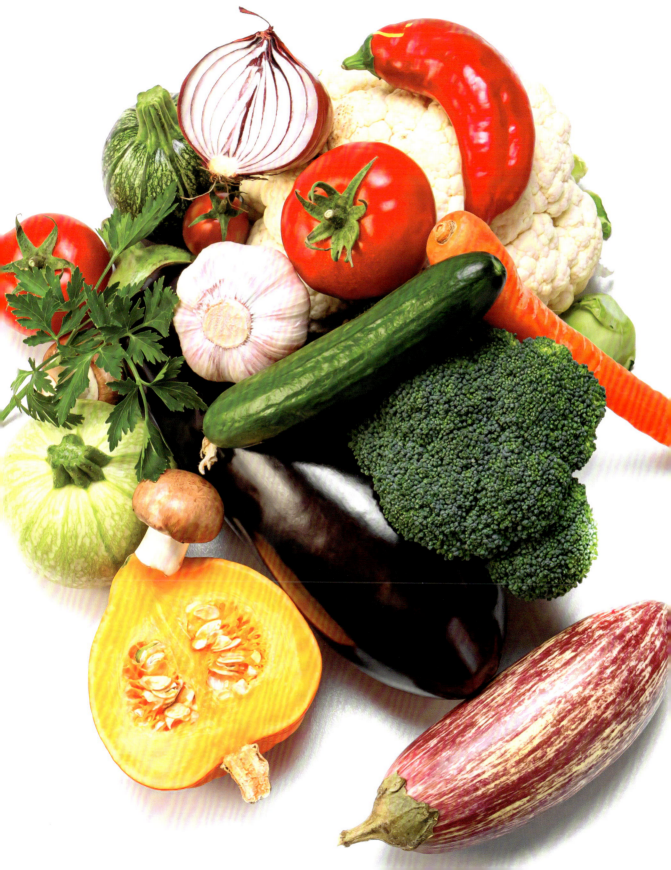

Some of this is a natural part of getting older, but the biggest reason for this sluggishness is because we simply aren't moving as much as we used to. Now, we're sitting behind a desk instead of running on a basketball court—and as a result, we're not burning as many calories throughout the day.

Now let's talk about macronutrients, or "macros" for short. There are three macronutrients (or "main" nutrients) that your body needs: protein, carbohydrates, and fat. Everyone will need a slightly different percentage of macros based on their goals: fat loss, weight loss, weight gain, strength building, and so on.

Absent a nutritionist, you may want to start with a relatively even percentage:

▶ 34% protein
▶ 33% carbohydrates
▶ 33% fats

I switch up my macros depending on my workout for the day. Check out the charts to the right to see what that looks like for me.

I eat the highest percentages of protein on leg day and on rest days. On leg day I do my heaviest lifting and eat the most food; on rest days, I eat less food, but a high percentage of protein, which helps with muscle repair.

MILO'S PERSONAL PLAN

I switch up my macros depending on my workout for the day. Here's what this looks like for me.

DAYS OF THE WEEK	PROTEIN	CARBS	FATS
SUNDAY: **LEG DAY**	50%	35%	15%
MONDAY: **REST DAY**	50%	35%	15%
TUESDAY: **PUSHING DAY**	40%	40%	20%
WEDNESDAY: **PULLING DAY**	40%	40%	20%
THURSDAY: **REST DAY**	50%	35%	15%
FRIDAY: **TOTAL BODY MUSCULAR ENDURANCE**	40%	45%	15%
SATURDAY: **TOTAL BODY CARDIO**	35%	45%	20%

MEAL PLAN RECOVERY DAY

I'm not a bodybuilder, and neither are you. And you probably don't have time to weigh all your food. The easier approach: Use your hands to measure your serving sizes. That's how I do it, and it'll help you follow my recovery-day meal plan.

BREAKFAST (6:30 TO 7:00 A.M.)
Egg White, Turkey, and Veggie Scramble
8 egg whites
2 palm-sized turkey breasts
1 handful chopped onions
1 handful chopped mushrooms
1 handful chopped bell peppers (red, green, and orange)

SNACK (9:30 TO 10:00 A.M.)
Turkey-Veggie Lettuce Wrap
1 large leaf lettuce
1 palm-size turkey breast
1 handful chopped broccoli
1 handful chopped cucumber
1 handful chopped red cabbage
1 kiwi

LUNCH (12:30 TO 1:00 P.M.)
Salmon-Quinoa Salad
1 hand-sized piece of salmon (about 8.5 inches long)
8 handfuls of romaine or butter lettuce
1 handful quinoa
½ handful onions
1 handful chopped cucumber
1½ handfuls chopped kalamata olives
1 handful chopped bell peppers

SNACK (3:30 TO 4:00 P.M.)
1 large red delicious apple
1 kiwi
2 plums

DINNER (6:30 TO 7:00 P.M.)
Chicken-Veggie Bowl
1 hand-sized chicken breast
2 heaping handfuls broccoli
2 handfuls green beans
1 handful quinoa

SNACK (9:30 TO 10:00 P.M.)
Shrimp and Citrus Salad
2 heaping handfuls romaine or butter lettuce
3 hard-boiled egg whites
1 handful shrimp
1 handful chopped cucumber
1 large grapefruit
4 splashes balsamic vinegar

When we lift weights, we create small microtears in the muscle fibers; when the body repairs these fibers, the muscles become bigger and stronger. To fuel this repair, we need protein. Of the three macronutrients, protein contains the most amino acids—which you can think of as the building blocks of muscle.

I eat the highest percentage of carbohydrates on the days when I'm doing the most endurance work. Carbs are absorbed by the body more quickly than protein and fat, and therefore, they are the easiest macronutrient for your body to convert to fuel.

Fat is important, too—you need some fat to burn fat, after all—but protein and carbohydrates play a big role in the recovery process. After a workout, you should add one last lift: pull a carb-and-protein bar, trail mix, or shake out of your gym bag to help kick-start the process of replenishing your muscles with glycogen and serving them a mix of amino acids during your cooldown.

These macros are there to help with recovery as much as they are to fuel our training. They become especially important as we age. As my good friend, Mark Smith, PhD, a nutritionist and the chief science officer for The Paleo Diet®, says: What we eat is the single biggest factor in our quality of life.

And when we focus on eating well and sleeping well, we can expect to recover faster from a workout, keep our energy levels up, and supercharge our immunity.

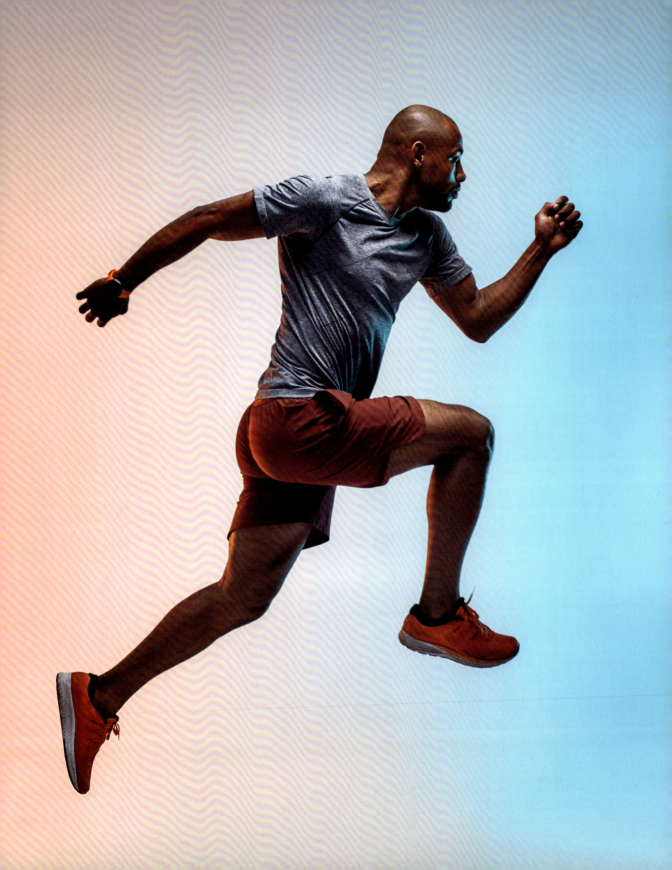

CHAPTER

04

TRAIN WITH NO PAIN

IN THIS CHAPTER, YOU'LL...

PROTECT YOURSELF FROM INJURY WITH THE WORLD'S BEST WARM-UP

—

BOOST MUSCLE GROWTH AND RECOVERY WITH MY THREE-STEP COOLDOWN

—

KEEP DOING WHAT YOU LOVE WITHOUT ACHES AND PAINS

THIS MAY be the most important chapter in the book. Even if you don't listen to anything else I've said, do this one thing: the warm-up. Specifically, the *dynamic* warm-up.

Now, I know what you're thinking: "Coach, I barely have time to fit in a workout, much less a warm-up." I know this because that's what almost *everyone* thinks. Most people view warm-ups as optional or even unimportant, the appetizer to the main course. I see this in the people I train. Knees don't lift high enough. Arms don't swing widely enough. Cores don't squeeze tight enough.

But hear me out.

For years, you've been told that you need to help your muscles recover after a workout. But the effort you put into priming your muscles for your workout is just as important. And you do this with a dynamic warm-up. You'll do more than touch your toes. We're trying to prep the body for everything it might encounter in your workout, so you'll move in a variety of directions, work quickly—and maybe break more of a sweat than you may expect. Warm up, and you'll prevent injuries and have a more productive workout, too.

Look, I get it: We're busy. We want to train—not prepare to train. The workout is the meat and potatoes; the warm-up is just a garnish. We always want the meat and potatoes.

The same goes for our workouts. We know the payoff from bench presses and biceps curls. They make us stronger and give us our "mirror muscles." Plus, we've done them a thousand times—why do we need to "get prepared" to do them again?

That type of thinking makes sense—but it's also the type of thinking that will set you up for an injury. Here's why: As we get older, our maximum heart rate decreases. That, in turn, decreases the amount of blood the heart pumps. Our lung

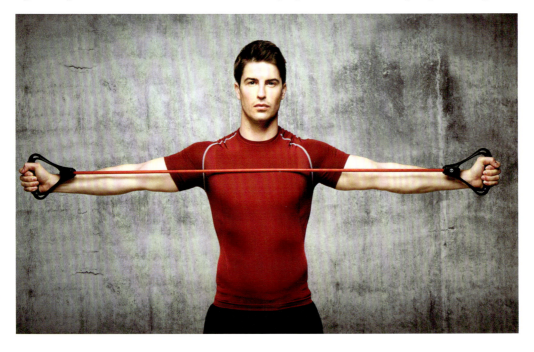

capacity decreases as well—we're not moving as much oxygen into the bloodstream, which also hinders our endurance. And when you have less blood and oxygen flowing to the brain, you can have slower reaction times. So making moment-to-moment decisions becomes a bit more of a challenge.

Some of this is inevitable, but a smart warm-up—one in which we're focused on each movement pattern—can help us combat that age-related decline.

I don't expect you to warm up for an hour or two. But at our age, we do not have the luxury of failing to prep for a workout.

So yes, that means you need to take the time to do this warm-up even if you only want to spend a half-hour curling dumbbells, and sure, this warm-up might actually take longer than your entire 10-minute run.

But you'd spend more than 10 minutes prepping for your daily meeting, right? And you spend more time getting dressed on date night, don't you? Your joints and muscles deserve that same attention. So make time for this warm-up. It's designed to bulletproof you for your workout—and prep your body for real life movement challenges, too.

WARM UP LIKE THE WORLD'S BEST ATHLETES

ONE OF THE BIGGEST lessons I've learned in my life as a trainer, especially when it comes to proper fitness, is to watch the best athletes in the world and break down what they do. Perhaps the best example of this occurred when I was sitting in the Bird's Nest, the nickname for Beijing National Stadium, at the Summer Olympics in 2008, watching Usain Bolt go through his 10-minute warm-up routine on the track.

I don't know what he did before he came onto the track. But even if he did nothing except that particular warm-up, this meant that he spent 10 minutes warming up so he could run a 9.69-second race, the 100-meter dash. Put another way, Bolt's warm-up was about 62 times longer than his (at that point) history-making sprint.

Bolt isn't an outlier, either. Let's study the NFL. Some of the players are on the field up to 2.5 hours before kickoff. First, they get on the field to acclimate to the temperature while wearing some gear. Some will break out foam rollers or bands. Others will have trainers with them, pushing them through a series of partner stretches, as well as skipping, shuffling, and hopping drills. They will do sprint mechanics—high knees, butt kicks, and A-skips. Then they go into the locker room for some hands-on therapy before putting on their gear and doing more mechanics. Then

comes the technique work that is specific to their individual positions. For some teams, all of that happens before the "team" warm-up. They don't spend the entire 2.5 hours moving, but they spend at least an hour warming up.

Now let's look at how many minutes one of those athletes might play in a game. If we assume that the player goes in for every offensive or defensive play (and there are very few players who do), he'll probably play an average of 65 downs a game. The average play only lasts 8 seconds or less, but for argument's sake, let's bump it up to 10 seconds. If our player goes in for 65 plays, for 10 seconds at a time, that means he's doing about 11 minutes worth of full-speed action—about $\frac{1}{15}$ of the time he spent warming up.

I realize you're not trying to run past 300-pound defenders or set land-speed records. But you have an older body than those pros, so the work you are planning to put in may be just as challenging. And remember: I'm not asking for hours upon hours of warm-up. All I want from you: 15 minutes. But to perform at your highest level in the gym, on the court, or anywhere else, you need to grant yourself 15 minutes to prepare for movement. It'll save you from injury and give your body the best chance possible to be great.

THE
WARM-UP

Perform this warm-up before each of your workouts.
It should take about 15 minutes. I do each of the
31 exercises listed below every day and twice on days
I work out or compete in some sporting event.

01 02 03

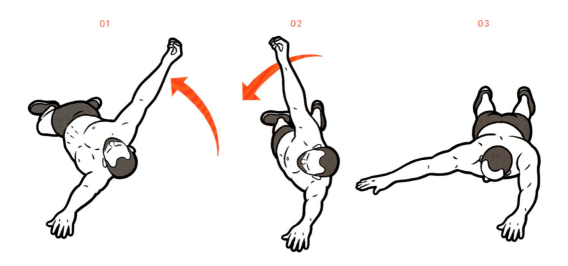

ROLLING PATTERNS

This total-body rolling series preps your body to rotate from left to right and right to left. Do 1 rep of each pattern.

SUPINE TO PRONE:
UPPER BODY REACH

▶ Lie faceup with your arms overhead and your feet hip-width apart. Keeping your right arm extended (1), stretch your right arm over your left shoulder, then roll left, leading with your upper body (2). You'll end up facedown, arms extended (3). Reverse the movement to return to your back.

▶ Repeat this movement on the right side.

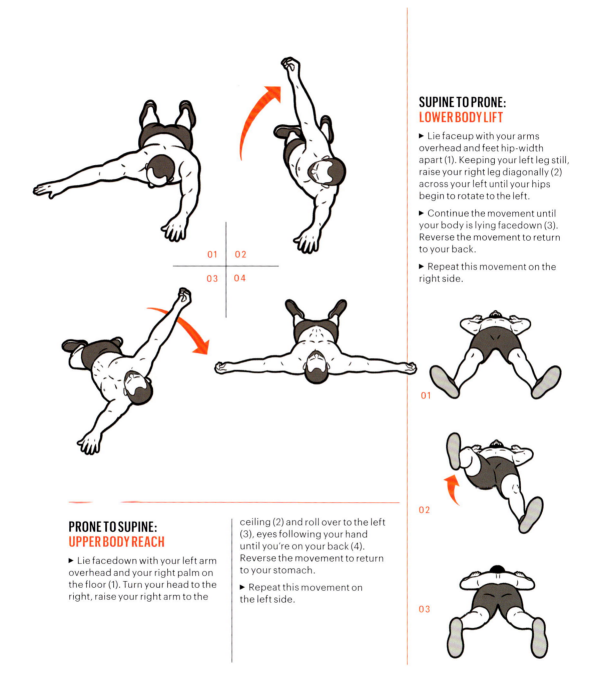

01 | 02
03 | 04

SUPINE TO PRONE:
LOWER BODY LIFT

▶ Lie faceup with your arms overhead and feet hip-width apart (1). Keeping your left leg still, raise your right leg diagonally (2) across your left until your hips begin to rotate to the left.

▶ Continue the movement until your body is lying facedown (3). Reverse the movement to return to your back.

▶ Repeat this movement on the right side.

01

02

03

PRONE TO SUPINE:
UPPER BODY REACH

▶ Lie facedown with your left arm overhead and your right palm on the floor (1). Turn your head to the right, raise your right arm to the ceiling (2) and roll over to the left (3), eyes following your hand until you're on your back (4). Reverse the movement to return to your stomach.

▶ Repeat this movement on the left side.

PRONE TO SUPINE:
LOWER BODY LIFT

▶ Lie facedown with your arms overhead and your feet hip-width apart (1). Keeping your left leg still, raise your right leg toward the ceiling and to the left. Your hips will begin to rotate (2). As you rotate your lower body, your upper body will follow (3).

▶ Continue to rotate your body until you're lying faceup (4).

Reverse the movement to return to your stomach.

▶ Repeat this movement on the left side.

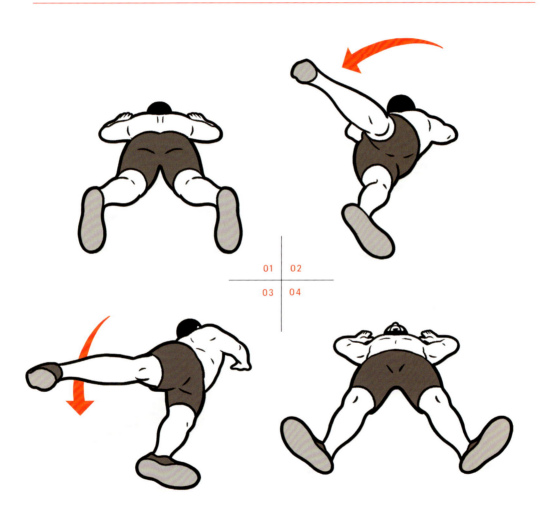

01	02
03	04

CRAWLING

Crawling may seem simple, but this crisscrossing movement pattern challenges your mind as much as your body.

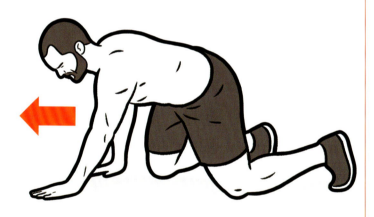

REVERSE CRAWL

▶ Start on all fours with your wrists directly below your shoulders and your knees positioned beneath your hips. Shift your knees shoulder-width apart. Brace your core and move backward, moving your right hand and left leg together, and left hand and right leg together (1).

▶ Alternating sides (2), use this movement pattern to keep crawling backward 10 steps per side.

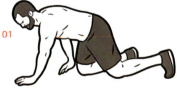

01

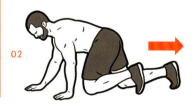

02

FORWARD CRAWL

▶ Start on all fours with your wrists directly below your shoulders and your knees positioned beneath your hips. Shift your knees shoulder-width apart. Brace your core and move forward, moving your right hand and left leg together, and left hand and right leg together.

▶ Using this movement pattern, keep crawling forward 10 steps per side. Want an added challenge? Hold a tennis ball or baseball between your chin and clavicle; this will force your head to rotate to one side as you crawl.

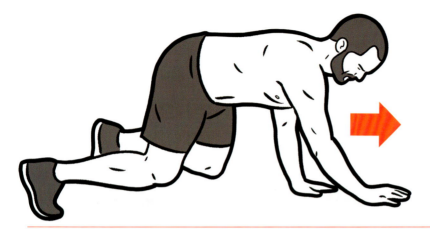

BEAR CRAWL

▶ Start on all fours with your wrists directly below your shoulders and your knees positioned beneath your hips. Shift your knees shoulder-width apart. Lift your knees one inch off the ground.

Brace your core and move forward, moving your right hand and left leg together, and left hand and right leg together.

▶ Using this movement pattern, keep crawling forward 10 steps per side.

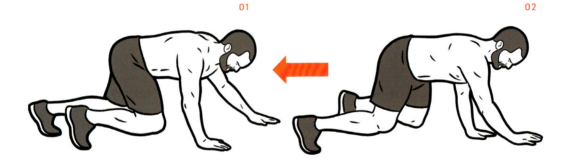

01

02

REVERSE BEAR CRAWL

▶ Start on all fours with your wrists directly below your shoulders and your knees positioned beneath your hips. Shift your knees shoulder-width apart. Lift your knees one inch off the ground. Brace your core and move

backward, moving your right hand and left leg together (1), and left hand and right leg together (2).

▶ Using this movement pattern, keep crawling backward 10 steps per side.

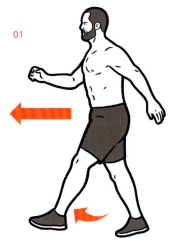

01

02

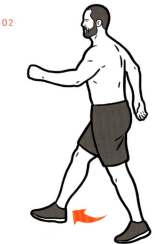

FORWARD SKIP

This exercise still utilizes the crisscross pattern of movement, while incorporating more cardio.

▶ Stand up straight with your hands at your sides and take one step forward with your right foot. With the right foot planted, swing your left foot and your right arm forward, and hop with the right foot (1).

▶ Continue the movement with the opposite foot and arm (2) for 10 hops per leg.

THE ONE EXERCISE YOU SHOULD STOP DOING WHEN YOU'RE OVER 40... AND WHAT TO DO INSTEAD

I ALWAYS TELL FOLKS THAT they can do any exercise they want as long as they do it with the correct intention and form. Weighted dips, Turkish getups, one-handed pullups—fine with me.

The exception to this rule: Long-distance running. Running farther than a mile just isn't the best use of your time. Focus on running harder over much shorter distances, because yes, your body can get a workout from even 50- or 100-meter sprints.

Before the National Coalition of Jogging Warriors runs me over with their Air Endorphin Zoom Ultra Pros, let me explain. There are only two reasons to jog, IMHO:

1. Jogging enables you to reach an ethereal oneness with the universe and puts you on a celestial plane to inner omnipotence.

2. You compete in long-distance running events.

That's it.

What's wrong with jogging, you ask? Everything, I would argue. In my experience, joggers have more injuries than any other group of people I work with. I have seen way too many of them come into my gym with stress fractures, shin splints, and joint damage. They've spent years or decades pushing through a nagging pain in their knee, wearing out their cartilage in the meantime, all to eke out a last mile or two.

You probably never gave your knee joint a second thought when you were 20. That changes when you get older. Statistics show that osteoarthritis typically appears in people over the age of 50, but I've seen people show signs of osteoarthritis in their 30s.

If you want to keep running in some capacity, do your body a favor and switch to sprinting. Your joints will thank you. Try this sprint workout at your local track twice a week: Run 100 meters. Rest 90 seconds (yes, that long). Repeat 6 times.

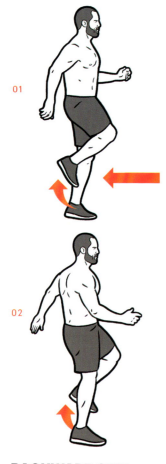

01

02

BACKWARD SKIP

The backward skip utilizes the crisscross pattern of movement, but requires more coordination than the forward skip.

▶ Stand up straight with your hands at your sides and take one step backward with your right foot. With the right foot planted, swing your left foot backward and your right arm backward and hop with the right foot (1).

▶ Continue the movement with the opposite foot (2) and arm for 10 hops per leg.

SINGLE-LEG HOP

The single-leg hop prepares your body to handle more explosive activities. It's especially good for athletes, who frequently perform movements while balanced on one foot, while their arms and other foot are in motion.

▶ Start in a standing position and shift your weight to your left foot. Bring your right knee up and bend your left arm behind you (as if in a running position) (1).

▶ Bend your left knee and hop forward. Land on the ball of your left foot (2). Quickly leap forward again with the same foot. That's 1 rep. Do 10, then repeat on the other leg.

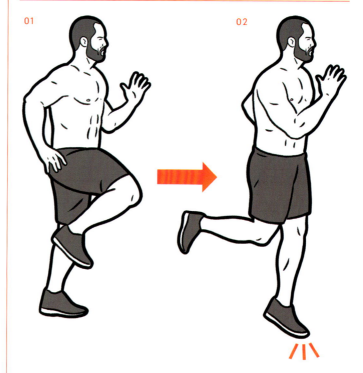

01

02

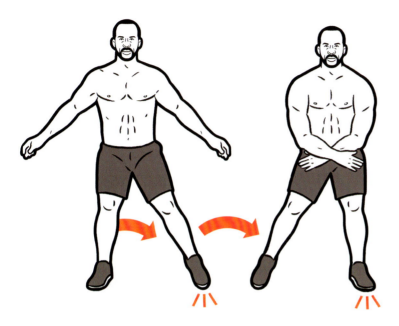

HIGH KNEE

This exercise prepares your body for explosive movements while running in a straight line.

▶ Run forward 20 steps, lifting your knees so your thighs are at least parallel to the ground on every stride.

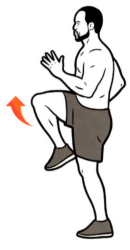

SHUFFLE

This exercise prepares you to shift your bodyweight laterally while in motion.

▶ Stand up straight, with your arms at your sides.

▶ Next, shifting your weight to your left foot, push off the ground and take a large hop to the right with your right foot. Quickly shuffle your left foot so it's beside your right foot, then take another hop with your right foot. Allow your arms to swing naturally and crisscross in front of your body.

▶ Repeat the pattern until you've done 10 shuffles. Repeat on the left side.

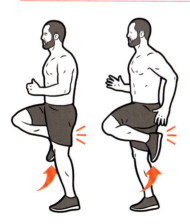

BUTT KICK

This exercise primes your hamstrings for explosive movements.

▶ Run forward 20 steps. On each stride, lift your knees high and touch your glute with your heel.

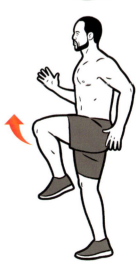

A-SKIP

This exercise prepares your body for high-intensity and explosive rhythmic movements.

▶ Stand tall. Pushing up off the ground with your left leg, lift your right knee up at a 90-degree angle while bending your left arm as if you were sprinting. Your thigh should be above parallel to the ground. Your left foot will take a little double hop forward (1).

▶ As the ball of your right foot lands, repeat the movement while lifting your left leg and right arm (2). Continue to alternate legs for 20 total steps.

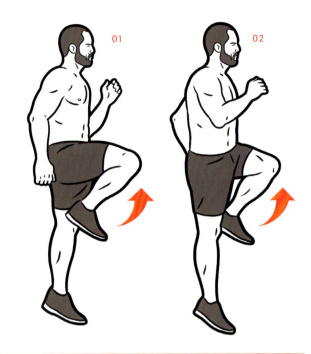

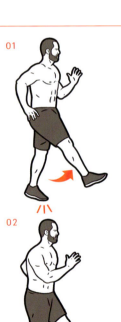

STIFF-LEGGED RUN

This exercise prepares your body to generate more horizontal force.

▶ Start in a standing position. Begin to run forward, but keep your legs almost completely straight as you do (1). As you lift each leg off the ground, flex your foot. As it hits the ground, try to drive the ground away and squeeze your glute. Alternate sides (2) until you've taken 20 total steps.

STIFF-LEGGED BOUND WITH ALTERNATE LEG

This exercise prepares the body to generate more horizontal force.

▶ Stand tall with your hands at your sides. Without bending your right knee, take a step forward with your left foot.

▶ Next, lift your right knee up high while you pull your foot in toward your groin, as if you're trying to hit your glute with your right heel. Then extend your right knee so your leg is straight and your ankle is flexed. Your right heel will strike the ground. Your arms should bend (as if you were sprinting) in coordination with the opposite foot. Take a few steps, then lift your left knee.

▶ Continue to alternate legs for 10 yards.

WALKING HAMSTRING

This exercise helps your body hinge at the hips.

▶ Stand with your arms at your sides. Take a small step forward with your right foot so that your right knee is extended. There should be a slight bend at the left knee (1).

▶ Keeping your spine neutral, push your butt back and lower your torso, stretching your right hamstring and both calves (2). Take three steps forward to shake out your legs, and repeat the process. (Don't skip the shakeout. Let that be a mental exercise.) Repeat the process for 5–7 reps per leg.

01

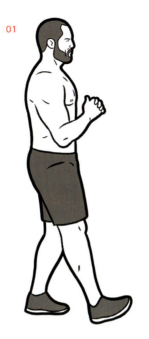

02

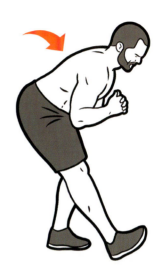

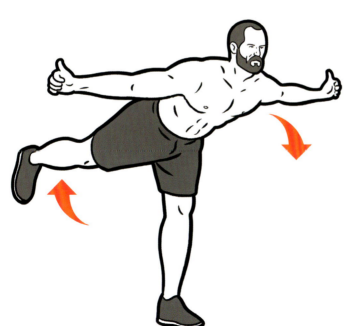

WALKING INVERTED HAMSTRING

This exercise prepares your body to hinge at the hips and improves your ability to balance on one foot.

▶ Stand with your arms extended out to your sides. Your left knee should bend slightly—no more than 5 degrees.

▶ Push your butt back, lowering your torso until it's parallel with the ground. Lift your right foot backward and up as you do this; your torso and right leg should form a straight line from head to heel. Hold for a moment, then lower your right leg to the starting position.

▶ Walk three steps forward, shake out your legs, and repeat the process with your left leg raised. Do 5–7 reps per side.

WALKING LEG KICK

This exercise preps your body for intense hip mobility on one side and higher-level stability on the other side.

▶ Stand tall. Take a step forward with your right foot (1). Moving from the hip, kick your left leg up as high as possible while keeping your right foot planted fully on the ground (2).

▶ Allow your left leg to swing back down until it is parallel with your right leg and allow it to flex (you should feel a quick stretch in your quads) (3).

▶ Repeat the process with your left leg stepping forward and your right leg kicking, alternating legs for 10 total reps.

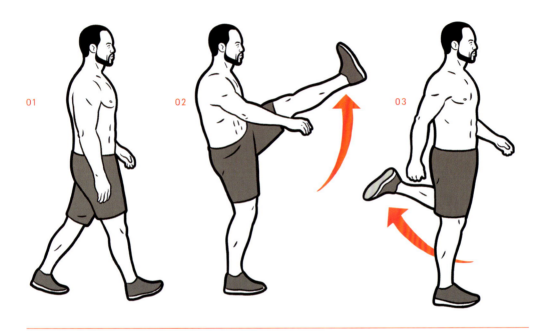

SPIDERMAN LUNGE

A variation of the classic lunge, this exercise is particularly good at boosting your hip mobility and stability.

▶ Start in the pushup position, hands directly below your shoulders, abs and glutes tight. Then step your left leg forward so it's alongside your left hand and your knee forms a 90-degree angle. Squeeze your right glute as you do this, and hold for a second.

▶ Shift back to the pushup position. Repeat the process on each side. Do 5 reps per leg.

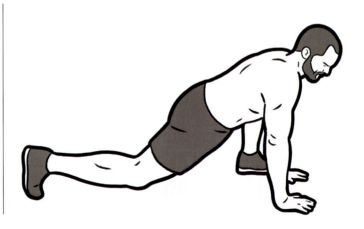

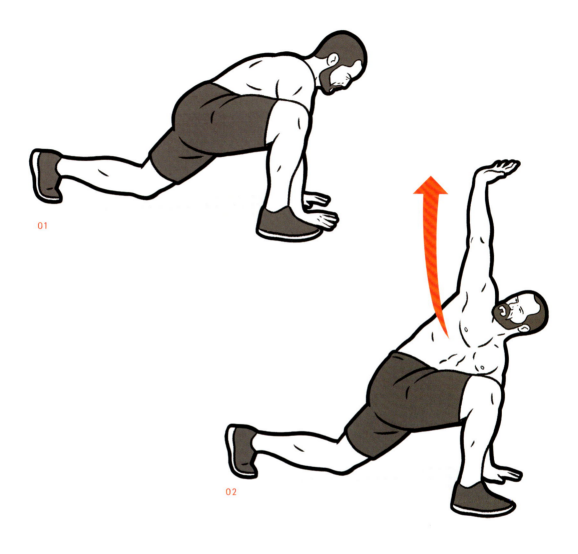

SPIDERMAN LUNGE
WITH ROTATION

This exercise adds an extra mobility movement to the Spiderman Lunge.

▶ Start in pushup position, hands directly below your shoulders, abs and glutes tight. Then step your right leg forward so it's alongside your right hand and your knee forms a 90-degree angle. Squeeze your left glute as you do this (1).

▶ Keeping your left hand on the ground, reach your right hand toward the ceiling, continuing to keep your hips square. Your eyes should follow your right hand (2). Reverse the movements back to pushup position, then repeat on the other side. Do 5 reps per leg.

LUNGE WITH OVERHEAD REACH

This exercise boosts mobility and stability.

▶ Start in a standing position, feet shoulder-width apart. Step forward with your left foot, lowering your body into a lunge.

▶ Drop your right knee as close to the ground as possible and press your arms toward the ceiling with your palms facing up. Stretch your torso for 5 seconds.

▶ Using your left heel, push your body back up to the starting position, lowering your arms back to your sides. Take three steps forward, and repeat on the other side. Do 5 reps per leg.

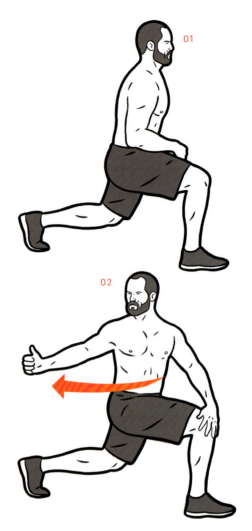

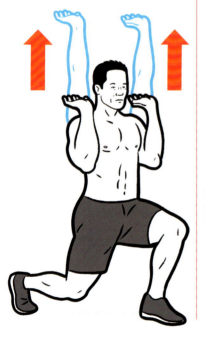

LUNGE WITH TWIST

This mobility exercise boosts mobility and stability while rotating your torso.

▶ Start standing, feet shoulder-width apart and hands at your sides. Step forward with your right foot, lowering your body into a lunge (1).

▶ Drop your left knee as close to the ground as possible. Then rotate your torso to the right, placing your left hand on the outside of your right knee to help deepen the rotation (2), and hold the position for a second.

▶ Using your right heel, push your body back to the starting position, returning your hands to your sides. Take three steps forward, then repeat on the other side. Do 5 reps per leg.

WALKING QUADRICEPS WITH OVERHEAD PRESS

This exercise boosts your single-leg stability and your quad and hip flexor stability.

▶ Stand with your feet shoulder-width apart and your hands at your sides. Lift your left leg behind you, grasp the top of your foot with your left hand and pull your heel into your glutes, keeping your thighs as parallel to each other as you can.

▶ Reach your right arm over your head as far as possible, keeping your palm facing the sky.

▶ Return to the starting position and repeat on the other side. Do 10 reps per leg.

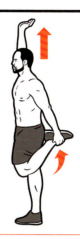

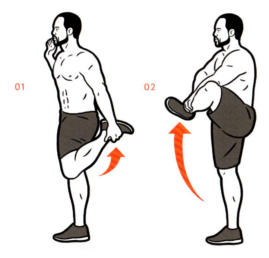

01   02

WALKING QUAD-TO-GLUTE WITH OVERHEAD PRESS

This exercise boosts your ability to balance on one leg and builds quad and hip flexor stability.

▶ Stand with your feet shoulder-width apart and your hands at your sides. Then, lift your left leg behind you and grasp the top of your foot with your left hand, pulling your heel into your glutes. Keep your thighs parallel to each other if you can.

▶ Extend your right arm over your head as far as possible, keeping your palm facing the sky (1).

▶ Let go of your left ankle and bring your left knee forward. Then grasp your left leg just above the ankle with your hands, pulling your shin toward your chest (2).

▶ Return your left leg to the starting position, then take three steps and repeat the movement on the other side. Do 5 reps per leg.

WALKING GLUTE

This exercise boosts your ability to balance on one leg and primes your glutes and hip sockets for more dynamic movements.

▶ Stand with your hands at your sides, then lift your right leg in front of your body.

▶ Raise your right leg by grasping just above your right ankle with your left hand. With your right hand, grab the shin a few inches above your left hand (1). Pull your shin toward your chest (2).

▶ Return to the starting position, then take three steps forward and shake out the leg. Repeat on the other side. Do 5 reps per leg.

01   02

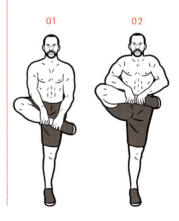

01

02

03

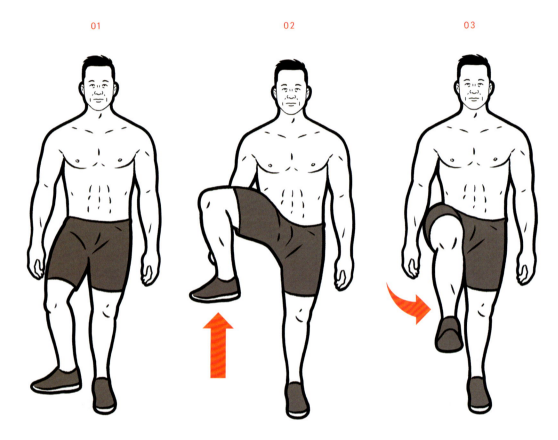

INTERNAL TO EXTERNAL HIP ROTATION

This exercise boosts your lower body mobility, particularly in your hips.

MOVING FORWARD

▶ Stand tall. Keeping your torso braced, turn your right foot to the right so your knee faces outward (1). Then raise your right knee so your thigh is parallel to the ground (2). Flex your hip and rotate your knee forward so it's in front of your torso (3), then place your foot on the ground. Repeat on the other side; do 10 reps per leg.

MOVING BACKWARD

▶ Stand tall. Keeping your torso braced, raise your right knee in front of you so your thigh is parallel to the ground (3). Keeping your knee bent, rotate your leg out to the right (2). Place your right foot on the ground (1), rotating it so both thighs are parallel. Repeat with the other leg. Do 10 reps per leg.

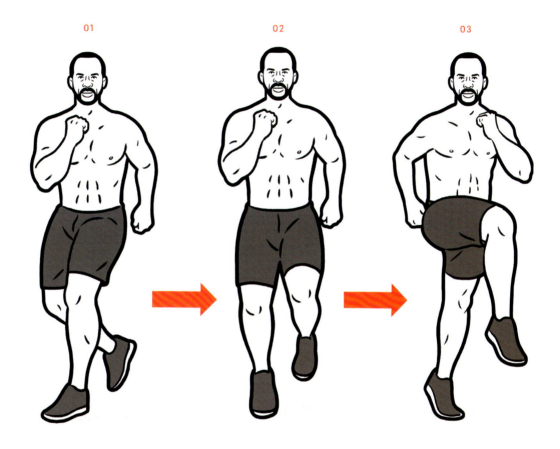

01 02 03

CARIOCA

This exercise will help build hip mobility and lower body explosiveness.

▶ You will move to the left as you run. Stand upright with your arms bent as if in a running position.

Twist your hips to the right and take a step back with your right foot so your right foot and leg are behind your left foot (1). This is the start.

▶ Take a step to the left with your left leg, then drive your right leg across your body, lifting your thigh high as you do. When your right

foot lands, immediately step to the left with your left leg again (2), then take another crossover step with your right leg. Continue doing this until you've taken 10 crossover steps with your right leg (3), then repeat on the other side.

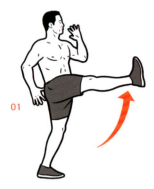

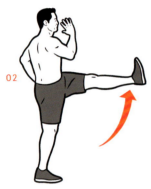

POWER SKIP

This exercise primes the body for explosive vertical movements.

▶ Stand in an upright position with your hands at your sides. Slightly flex your left knee then simultaneously and explosively push off the ground with your left leg and thrust your right knee toward the ceiling. Bend your left arm into a running position (as if you were pumping your arm during a sprint). Your right knee should be at a 90-degree angle (1). The goal is to jump vertically, not horizontally. Land on your left foot. Take a step forward with your right foot and, from a slightly flexed right knee, simultaneously push off the ground with your right foot and thrust your left knee (2). Repeat the movements for 10 yards.

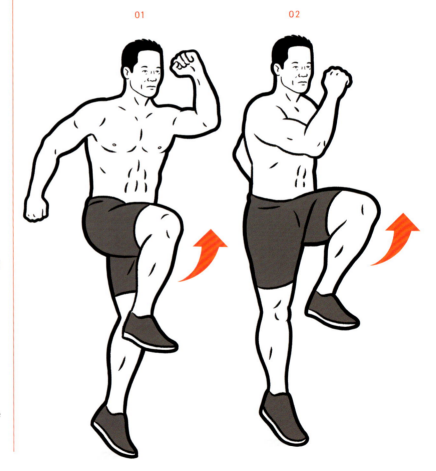

FRANKIE SKIP

This prepares your body for explosive movements that recruit your hips.

▶ Stand with your arms at your sides. Skip forward by pushing off the ground with your left foot while swinging your right leg forward from the hip. Your right leg, while remaining straight, should reach at least parallel to the ground and your left hand should be about as high as your face. Your left foot will give a little hop just like you did during the A-Skip (1).

▶ As the ball of your right foot lands, repeat the movement while lifting your left leg and right arm (2). Continue to alternate legs for 10 yards.

YOUR
THREE-STEP COOLDOWN

TWO DECADES AGO, when you were done with your workout, you were, well, done with your workout. Now, if you want your over-40 body to bounce back from workouts optimally, you need to give it some help. That means making smart nutrition choices and logging a bit more movement.

STEP ONE:
MOVE A LITTLE MORE

I took martial arts classes decades ago. Our sensei would not let us leave the dojo until we had a proper cooldown. He'd tell us that we had to "reinforce the training and reinforce the skill."

At the time, I didn't completely understand it. All I knew was that he had badass skills and I wanted badass skills. But his message always stuck with me. Today, however, there is research that supports his advice—namely, that stretching helps a process called post-exercise anabolic signaling, during which the body builds muscle.

Basically, your cooldown stretching can boost your ability to grow muscle—and that's important because, as I mentioned earlier, you already lose muscle as you age. That's why doing a cooldown after every workout is so important; it just may spark more muscle-building than all those post-lift protein shakes. Plus, these movements are proven to benefit your body, pushing you into positions you should always be capable of reaching and stimulating easy bloodflow.

Don't worry, though: It won't take long. Just do one rep of each of these seven exercises. (And here's a bonus: If you absolutely can't do a full warm-up, you can use these moves as a lightning-fast warm-up too. If you're going to do that, do five reps of each move.)

01. FLEX FORWARD

▶ Stand, arms hanging by your sides. Push your butt back and lower your torso, bending forward at the hips and touching your toes (or lowering as far as you can). Hold for 5 seconds. Return to the starting position.

02. EXTEND BACKWARD

▶ Stand with your arms above your head. Bend as far backward as possible while keeping your feet planted. Return to the starting position.

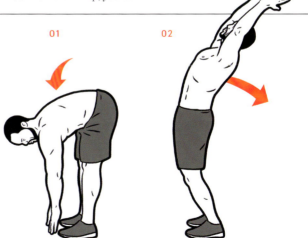

01   02

03. ROTATE LEFT AND RIGHT

▶ Stand with your feet together, toes pointing forward, arms hanging by your sides. Turn your body to the left as far as possible while keeping your toes facing forward. Return to the starting position and repeat on the other side.

04. BALANCE ON YOUR LEFT FOOT (AND YOUR RIGHT)

▶ Stand tall with both feet together. Lift your left leg until your knee forms a 90-degree angle and your thigh is parallel to the ground. Hold that position for 10 seconds, keeping your hips and shoulders square to the front. Return to the starting position and repeat on the other side.

05. SQUAT

▶ Stand with your feet shoulder-width apart, arms held in front of you. Keeping your abs tight, push your butt back and bend your knees, allowing your torso to descend. Lower as far as you can. Return to the starting position.

STEP TWO:
CARB UP (YES, REALLY)

Now that you're done sweating, it's time to eat. But don't start by focusing on protein. Instead, focus on carbs. I know what you've been told about carbs, but it's simply not true. Carbs aren't the enemy. Instead, they play a critical role in helping you recover fully from your workout so you can hit the gym again tomorrow with the same intensity you did today.

That's because your body's levels of glycogen (i.e., stored carbohydrates) drop after a workout. In order to kick-start the process of rebuilding your muscles, you'll need to replenish those stores with more carbohydrates. (If you have diabetes, your carb intake may be different; talk to your doctor before making any changes to your diet.)

The ideal time to replenish your glycogen levels is after a workout. That's because after exercise, your muscle cells are more sensitive to insulin, a

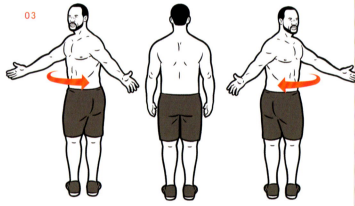

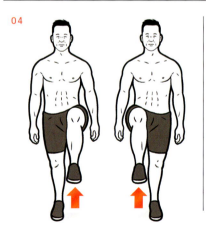

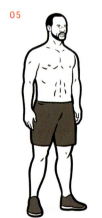

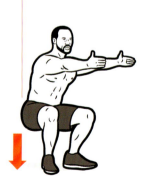

hormone that helps move glucose (a simple carbohydrate) into your blood, where it can be stored as energy.

Now that the cells are open to receive more glucose, it's your job to give it to them.

What kind of food should you eat? Right after a workout, I like to eat fruit, which is a source of glucose, healthy carbs, and fiber (check out some of my favorites in the chart to the right).

I choose fruits that have a lower glycemic load (GL). This is a number that a food is assigned based on how quickly it makes your blood sugar levels rise, while also taking into account the amount of carbohydrates it contains per serving. The higher a food's number, the faster it will raise your blood sugar.

The GL differs from the glycemic index (GI), which assigns a food a numeric score based only on how quickly that food increases blood sugar levels. Pure glucose (sugar) for example, has a score of 100, whereas foods with low scores tend to contain more fiber and fat.

I like using the GL much more than the GI because it accounts for not just the quality of the food but also the quantity of the food. Some carbs tend to get a bad rap with the GI. Watermelon, for example, has a high GI, but you'd have to eat a ton of it before it would be unhealthy.

A single serving of food with a GL of more than 20 is considered high. Aim for foods that have GL scores of 10 or less after your workouts. The chart below breaks down a few of my favorites.

THE BEST FRUITS TO EAT POST-WORKOUT

Low-GL fruits won't cause a spike in your blood sugar, making them a great recovery food. Below are my go-to snacks.*

FRUIT	SERVING SIZE	GLYCEMIC LOAD (GL)
PLUM	2 large	2
GRAPEFRUIT	1 large	3
PEAR	2 medium	4
KIWI	2 large	5
APPLE	1 large	5

Keep in mind that this is just one post-recovery snack, though. Depending on how intense your workout is, it may take you up to 48 hours to completely replenish your muscle glycogen, and that's if you're eating a healthy amount of carbohydrates.

STEP THREE:
HAVE SOME PROTEIN

No, I didn't forget about protein, but it plays a smaller role in your over-40 post-lift regimen

than you may think. Yes, protein helps us build muscle cells. But research has shown that folks who take post-resistance-training protein supplements see a reduction in the effect of the supplements as they grow older. I constantly look at quality over quantity, aiming to get my protein from the best sources, and chasing natural sources of protein over shakes and bars.

That's especially important once the workout is done, when your muscles are spent. So aim for 25 to 30 grams of protein, and aim to get it not from shakes, but from foods like chicken, salmon, beef, or eggs.

Enjoy this post-workout meal, too! Your muscles put in work. Now, you're feeding them.

*Serving sizes are based on what I typically consume as a 218-pound, 6-foot man.

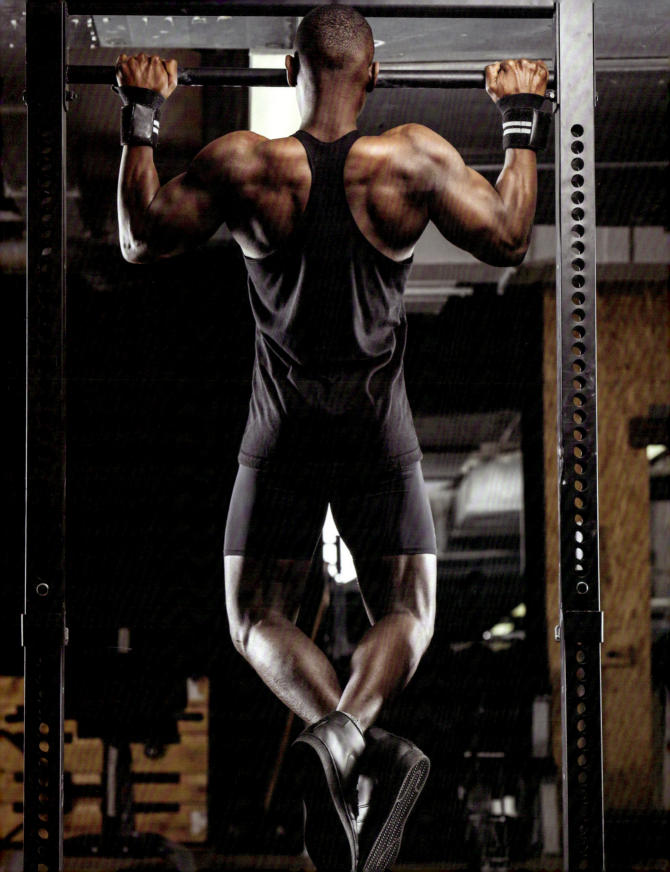

CHAPTER

05

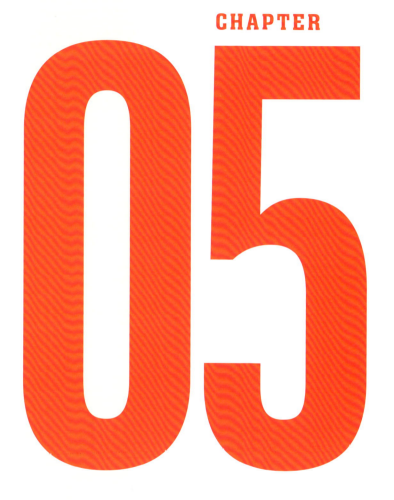

IN THIS CHAPTER, YOU'LL...

ELIMINATE JOINT PAIN HEAD TO TOE

MAINTAIN MOBILITY SO YOU NEVER HAVE TO SLOW DOWN

BUILD A FOUNDATION THAT WILL SHIELD YOU FROM INJURY

BULLETPROOF
YOUR JOINTS

I'LL NEVER forget the first time a doctor told me I had "old shoulders." I was 43 years old, able to knock out sets of 20 reps of pullups with ease. One day I felt a crazy-deep, dull pain from the back of my left shoulder deep into my left lat. The pain was strange and worrisome, and I couldn't do a single pullup.

My physical therapist referred me for a nerve conduction study, which scared the hell out of me at the time, because I didn't know if the doctor would have to stick me with needles. (I absolutely hate needles.) But after 30 minutes of poking and prodding my shoulders, ankles, and knees, the doctor told me I was fine.

I must have given him a look that said, "Well, I sure don't *feel* fine," because the doctor said, "Mr. Bryant, you have 43-year-old shoulders. They're old and they're susceptible to wear and tear."

I left the doctor's office fuming (okay, pissed) and called a friend on the way home to vent. This friend asked me if I was still doing my Tom House exercises (more on Tom in a minute). Sure enough, I wasn't. Now I was even more pissed, but this time, I was mad at myself.

When I got home, I started doing these joint-strengthening exercises for five minutes a day, three times a week, and I haven't stopped doing them since. I've

never had another problem with my shoulders, traps, or lats.

When you were younger, you probably thought about your muscles a lot more than you thought about your joints. But I can assure you that they are equally important.

Your joints are the areas where two or more bones meet. Your knees (where your femur and tibia meet) and your shoulders (where your humerus and scapula meet) are just a few examples. Many of these bones also have cartilage on the ends of them, which helps them move and prevents them from rubbing into each other.

As we get older, some of us naturally lose cartilage, which makes it more difficult to move the joint without feeling pain. But we lose more cartilage and joint mobility because we stop using the joints the way we did 20 years ago. And when it comes to joint mobility, you either use it or lose it.

Take the Tom House shoulder circuit that I'm such a fan of. These exercises work all the little muscles in the shoulder capsule that help rotate the joint. By performing each movement pattern that the shoulders use— and by regularly moving the joint in those directions—you can maintain the joint's mobility and flexibility for years to come.

Put another way: We can bulletproof the joint.

BULLETPROOF
TOTAL BODY SERIES

Sure, some of these exercises may seem tedious, if not downright boring. But if we do them with as much energy and passion as we put into deadlifts and squats, our "old shoulders"—not to mention our backs, legs, core, arms, and every other part of our bodies—are going to be impregnable.

Do these exercises at least twice a week to keep your joints healthy. If you experience pain, you may need to do them more often (and see a movement specialist to identify the origin of the pain). These are movements your body is meant to do, so doing them frequently won't harm the muscles.

SHOULDERS

Without further ado, I present the Tom House exercises. They take their name from—you guessed it—Tom House, the ex-MLB pitcher who ran a sports sciences department at the University of Southern California and who has improved more NFL quarterbacks' throwing mechanics over the past decade than anyone else. House has spent his career working with guys like Hall of Fame pitcher Nolan Ryan, who threw a no-hitter at age 44. House's drills might not add serious juice to your fastball, but they'll prep your body to hang pain-free from jungle gyms, dominate backyard football games, and crush weight room shoulder presses.

Each of these movements requires you to turn your palms in three different directions, targeting each of the movement patterns that the shoulders must perform. Do each of these in order, four times per week.

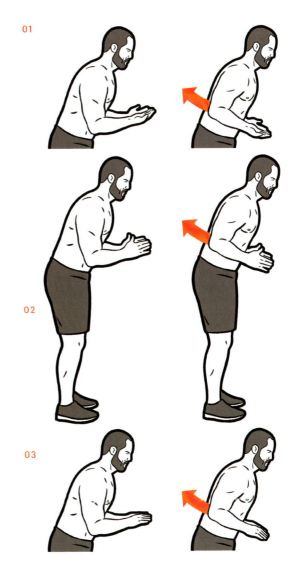

01

02

03

SAW

▶ Stand with your arms by your sides, your torso bent slightly forward, and your elbows bent at 90-degree angles. Without changing the angle of your forearms, rotate your palms so they're facing the ceiling and move them back and forth 10 times (as if you're sawing a piece of wood) (1).

▶ Next, rotate your hands so your palms are facing each other and repeat the movement 10 times (2).

▶ Rotate your hands so your palms are facing the ground and perform the movement 10 more times (3).

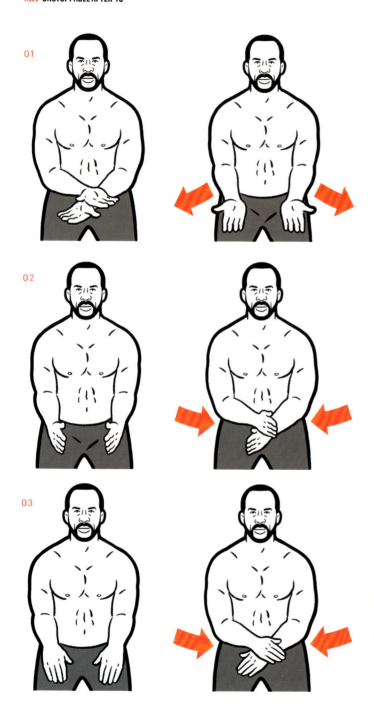

01

02

03

CRISSCROSS

▶ Stand with your upper arms pressed against your sides and your elbows bent at 90-degree angles. Push your butt back slightly so your torso bends forward a bit. Press your upper arms into your torso. This is the start.

▶ Rotate your palms so they're facing the ceiling and rapidly cross your hands in front of your body 10 times (your entire forearm will move as you do this) (1).

▶ Next, rotate your hands so your palms are facing each other and repeat the movement 10 times (2).

▶ Lastly, rotate your hands so your palms are facing the ground and repeat the movement 10 times (3).

CRADLE ROCK

▶ Stand with your upper arms next to your sides. Push your butt back and shift your torso forward slightly. Adjust your arms so they're just in front of your body, palms facing upward, elbows bent at 90-degree angles.

▶ Keeping your elbows flexed, spread your arms and bring your hands rapidly toward each other, rapidly passing your left hand under your right and vice versa. Do 10 reps per side (1).

▶ Next, rotate your hands so your palms are facing the ground and repeat the movement 10 times (2).

▶ Then rotate your hands so your palms face your body and do 10 more reps (3).

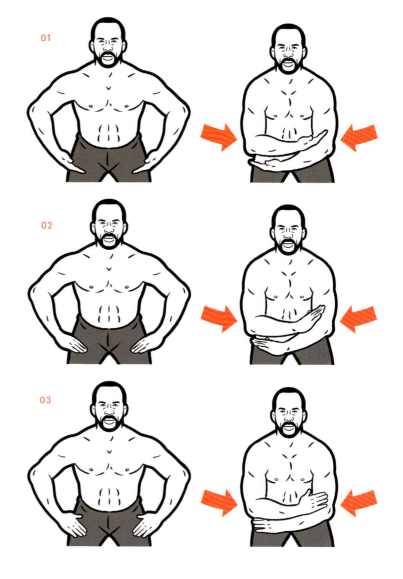

01

02

03

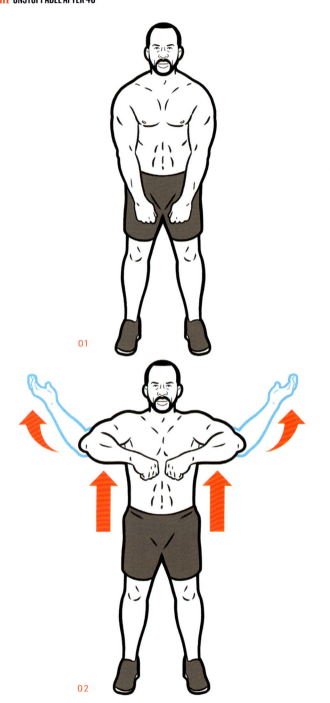

01

02

WHY ME

▶ Stand, then push your butt back and shift your torso forward slightly. Let your arms hang naturally near your thighs (1).

▶ Keeping your shoulder blades tight, pull your hands upward. As your hands reach chest height, rotate your shoulders back and open your elbows so your hands face forward—as if you're saying, "C'mon, why me?" (2)

▶ Return to the starting position and repeat for 10 reps.

SWIMMER

▶ Stand tall. Clasp your hands together in front of your chin, positioning one thumb pointing up and one thumb pointing down. Keeping a tight grip, pull on both hands without breaking the clasp. This is the start (1).

▶ Move your arms rapidly from side to side 10 times in each direction. Your arms should stay parallel to the ground throughout the movement. Return to the starting position (2).

▶ Do 10 forward circles with your arms, followed by 10 backward circles (3).

▶ Return to the starting position and rotate your shoulders and elbows as if you're swimming the forward crawl. Do this exercise for 10 reps, then rotate your shoulders and elbows and perform the exercise in reverse for 10 reps (4).

▶ Return to the starting position and try to squeeze your elbows and forearms together in front of your chest for 3 reps (5).

▶ Repeat this entire cycle with your hands clasped, but this time, pushing your hands together instead of pulling them apart.

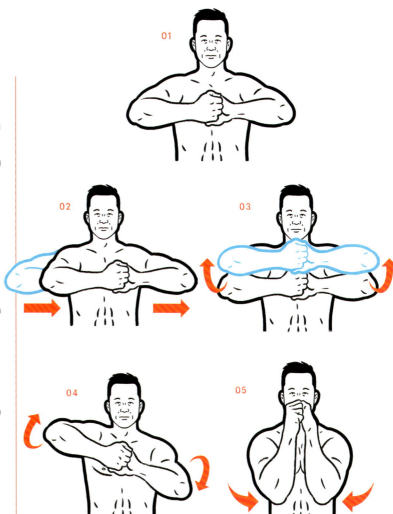

01

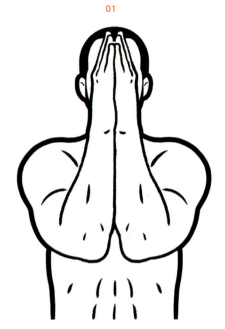

02

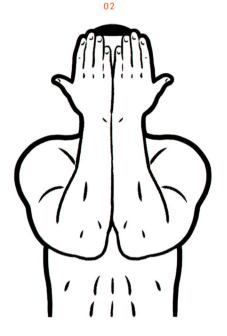

03

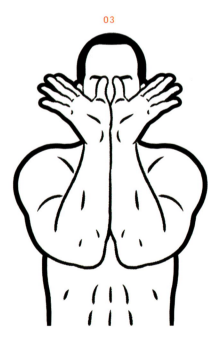

PRAYER

▶ Stand with your forearms in front of your chest. Your arms should be touching from the elbows to your fingertips, with your palms pressed together (as if you were praying). Squeeze your entire forearm, wrists, palms and fingers as hard as you can for 10 seconds (1).

▶ Next, turn your palms toward you, pressing your forearms together so your pinkies are touching. Squeeze as hard as you can for 10 seconds (2).

▶ Then, rotate your palms so that they're facing away from you, pressing your forearms together so your thumbs are touching. Squeeze as hard as you can for 10 seconds (3).

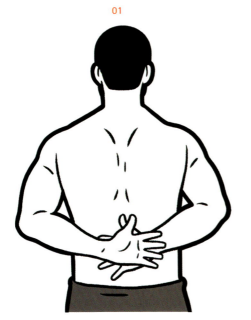

01

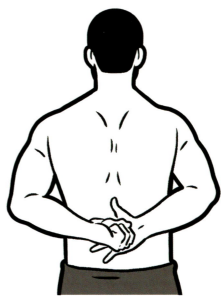

02

BACKSIDE PRESS

▶ Stand with both of your hands behind your back, just above your glutes.

▶ Put the back of your right hand against your lower back and open your palm (1). Then put the fist of your left hand on top of your right palm, pressing into it as hard as you can for 10 seconds.

▶ Rotate your left fist so that your left thumb is on your right palm (2). Press your fist in again as hard as you can for 10 seconds.

▶ Then, rotate your left fist so that the side of your left pinky finger is against your right palm (3). Press your fist in as hard as you can for 10 seconds.

▶ Allow the arms to relax, then repeat the process with the back of your left palm against your lower back and your right fist pressing into your left palm in all three positions.

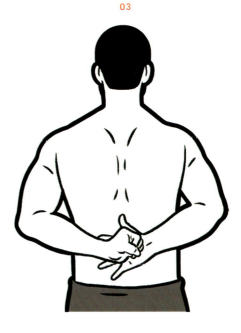

03

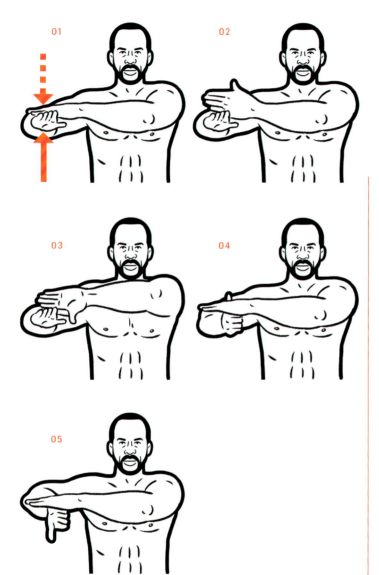

SHOULDER SQUARE

▶ Stand with your right arm raised to the side at shoulder height. Bend your elbow at a 90-degree angle, keeping your upper arm parallel with the ground. Take your left arm and raise it in front of your body, at shoulder height, and bend your arm at a 90-degree angle, keeping your arm parallel with the ground. Place your left hand on top of your right hand. Your arms should form a square.

▶ Press down with the left hand lightly while pressing up with the right hand lightly. Hold for 10 seconds (1).

▶ Rotate the left hand so that the thumb is pointing up. Press and hold for 10 seconds (2).

▶ Rotate the left hand so that the thumb is pointing down. Press and hold 10 seconds (3).

▶ Rotate the left hand so that the palm is flat and rotate the right hand so that the thumb points up. Press and hold for 10 seconds (4).

▶ Rotate the right hand so that the thumb is pointing down. Repeat the pressing pattern; hold for 10 seconds (5). Repeat the entire sequence to the other side.

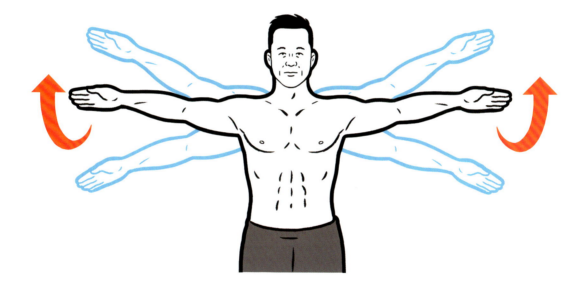

ARM CIRCLE

▶ From a standing position, stretch your arms out to your sides so they form a 20-degree angle with your torso. Rotate your hands so your palms are facing down and perform 10 small forward circles with your arms. Next, perform 10 circles with a slightly wider arc, followed by 10 circles with an arc that's even wider.

▶ Return to the starting position and rotate your hands so that your palms are facing forward away from your body. Then repeat the small, medium, and large circles for 10 sets each.

▶ Return to the starting position and rotate your palms so that they're facing down again, and perform 10 small backward arm circles, followed by 10 medium circles and 10 large circles.

ROTATOR CUFFS

All too often, I see people who work their shoulders but neglect their rotator cuffs. We do push-ups and pullups. Bench presses and incline bench presses. Lateral raises and bent-over rows.

And yet, many exercises (especially if they aren't done the right way) neglect to work the rotator cuff—a group of four small muscles around the shoulder joint that keep the joint functional. These muscles and tendons help you rotate, raise, and lower your arm. More importantly, they allow us to throw and reach and swing with efficiency.

There's no getting around it: If you want to bulletproof your shoulders, you'll need to fit rotator cuff exercises into your workout. Do these movements at least twice a week.

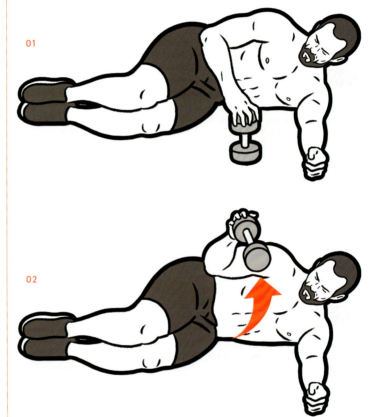

01

02

SIDE-LYING LATERAL ROTATION

▶ Holding a very light dumbbell in your right hand, lie on your left side with your right upper arm pressed against your torso and your elbow bent at a 90-degree angle (1).

▶ Keeping your elbow against your side, raise the dumbbell up; you'll feel your shoulder working (2). Hold for 2 seconds, then return to the starting position. Do 10 reps. Repeat with your left arm for 10 reps.

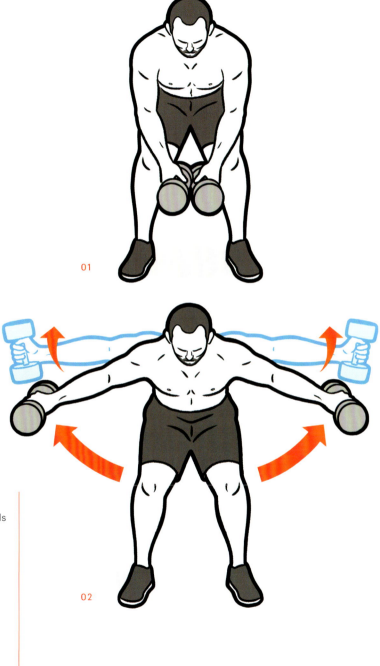

01

02

REVERSE FLY

▶ Stand holding light dumbbells in each hand. Bend your knees slightly and push your butt back, lowering your torso until it's nearly parallel with the ground. This is the start (1).

▶ Without moving your torso, raise your arms straight out to your sides. Squeeze your shoulder blades as you do this, and rotate your hands so your palms face forward (2). Lower; repeat for 10 reps.

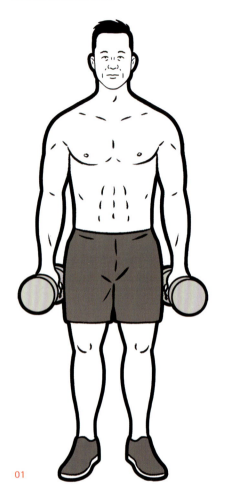

01

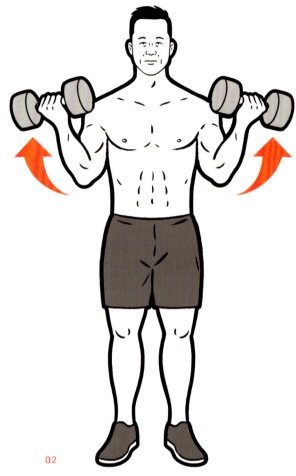

02

This exercise can be performed from a standing, sitting, or tall- or half-kneeling position.

PRECISION BICEPS CURL

▶ Stand holding light dumbbells in your hands, core and glutes tight (1).

▶ Curl the dumbbells upward, flexing your biceps. As you do this, rotate your arms out so that your forearms flare outward. Turn your palms to face your torso at the top of the curl (2). Pause, then slowly lower to the start. Repeat for 10 reps.

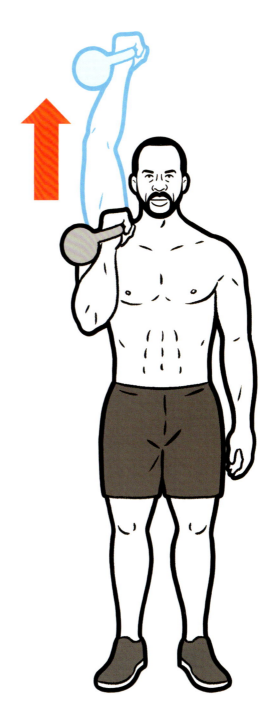

KETTLEBELL SHOULDER PRESS

▶ Stand upright and hold a kettlebell in your right hand in the rack position: right lat squeezed, elbow pulled toward your ribcage, forearm nearly perpendicular to the ground. Maintain tension in your wrist.

▶ Tighten your abs and glutes, and press the weight directly overhead. Return to the starting position. Do 10 reps. Repeat on the left side.

SPINE

My college strength coach, John Stucky, told me that people with good mobility in their hips and T-spine (the thoracic spine, or middle and upper spine) usually end up being pretty mobile athletes.

That's why I've spent so much time searching for movements that help boost my hip and spine mobility. (Many of these are included in the dynamic warm-ups I've already given you, too.)

But exercises that build thoracic spine mobility are more than warm-ups. They're moves that counteract the way life sabotages your over-40 body. We've all spent years hunched over our desks and texting on our smartphones, all of which has messed up our spines. I see so many people who don't do enough to open up their torso or rotate their thoracic spine, causing muscle imbalances that can lead to a condition called Upper Crossed Syndrome, or pain in the back of the neck and the spine between the lower shoulder blades.

Since I know you're not going to put down the phone or step away from the desk, perform 2 sets of each of these exercises at least 3 times per week.

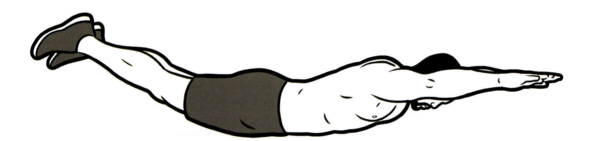

SUPERMAN HOLD

▶ Lie facedown on a flat, firm surface with your arms extended in front of you, legs extended behind you.

▶ Squeeze your glutes, raise your legs a few inches off the ground, and tighten your back muscles, raising your arms a few inches off the ground, as if flying like Superman. Hold for 5 seconds. Repeat 10 times.

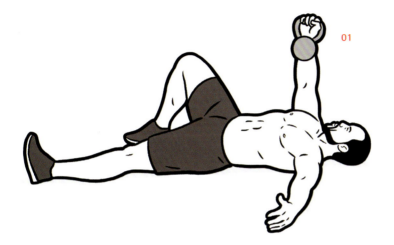

01

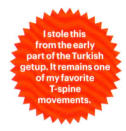

I stole this from the early part of the Turkish getup. It remains one of my favorite T-spine movements.

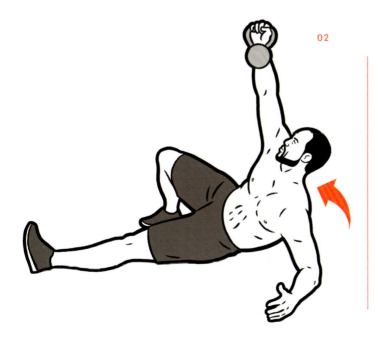

02

TWO-STEP GETUP

▶ Lie faceup with your left leg straight and your right knee bent, right foot flat on the ground. Your left arm should be on the ground. Hold a light dumbbell in your right hand, directly over your right shoulder (1).

▶ Pressing your left upper arm and elbow into the ground, push your right shoulder upward, continuing to keep your right arm straight. Watch the weight as you do this (2).

▶ Rise to a sitting position by straightening your left arm until your upper body is propped up only on your left hand. Lower with control back to the start. Do 10 reps per arm.

HIPS

You're sitting down while reading this, aren't you? Of course you are. We've been sitting for the past 20 years. And that sitting can lead to the dreaded...Dead Butt Syndrome. (Yes, it exists.)

The technical term for this syndrome is "gluteal amnesia," and contrary to its name, it's no laughing matter. Sitting for long periods of time can tighten the hip flexors, the muscles that help flex your hip, and weaken the gluteus medius, the glute muscle that helps stabilize the pelvis. Combine that weakness and tightness and you have a recipe for hip and lower back pain as well as a weak abdominal core.

To help reverse that damage, perform 2 sets of each of these exercises at least 3 times per week.

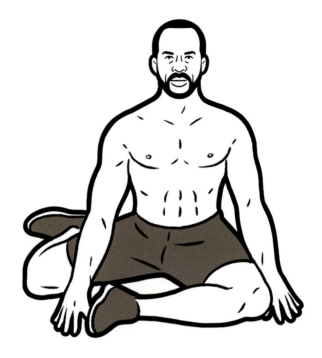

90/90

▶ Sit on the ground with your right leg in front of your body, your right knee bent at a 90-degree angle. Your left leg should be to the side, with the knee bent at a 90-degree angle pointing in the same direction as the right knee.

▶ Keeping your torso straight and your feet in place, rotate your knees so your left leg is in front of your body at a 90-degree angle and the right leg is out to the side at a 90-degree angle. Putting as much pressure on your right glute as you put on your left, trying to close the gap between the right side of the pelvis and the ground.

▶ Rotate side to side for 10 total reps.

90/90 WITH REAR LIFT

▶ Begin in the 90/90 starting position with the legs going to the right. Raise the rear foot off the ground while keeping the torso and pelvis stable. Perform 10 reps. Repeat on the other side.

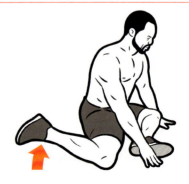

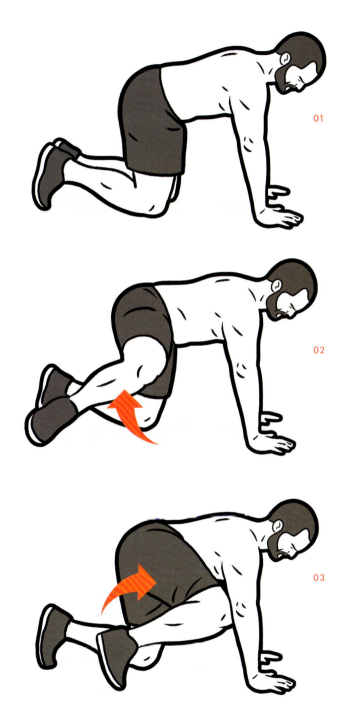

QUADRUPED HIP ROTATION

▶ Start on all fours, hands directly below shoulders, knees directly below hips (1).

▶ Keeping your hips stable and your knees bent at 90 degrees, raise your right leg until your thigh is nearly in line with your body. Rotate your knee out so it flares to the side, then bring it forward so that it's slightly in front of the left leg (2). Repeat the movement for 10 reps.

▶ Reverse the movement, bringing your right knee forward, then rotating it out to the side, before returning to the starting position for another 10 reps (3).

▶ Repeat the movements with your left leg.

COMERFORD HIP COMPLEX

This exercise, designed by Australian physical therapist Mark Comerford, consists of five different clamshell movements that strengthen your glutes. Do each one in the sequence for 10 reps before moving on to the next one. After you complete the circuit, roll over and repeat on the other side.

01. CLAMSHELL

▶ Lie on your left side with your knees bent at 45-degree angles. Your right leg should be stacked on top of your left leg and your knees and feet should be touching.

▶ Keeping your feet together, raise your right knee as high as you can without moving your hips. Hold for 3 seconds, then lower your right leg to the starting position.

02. REVERSE CLAMSHELL

▶ Start in the clamshell position, knees together. Keep the knees together and raise your right calf and foot a few inches off your left leg. Hold for 3 seconds, then lower your right leg to the starting position.

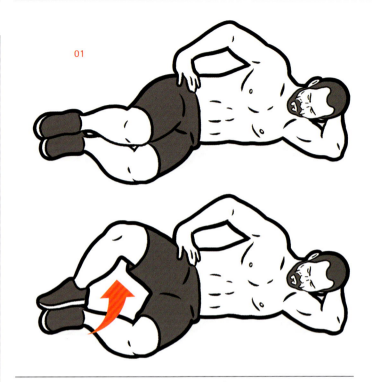

01

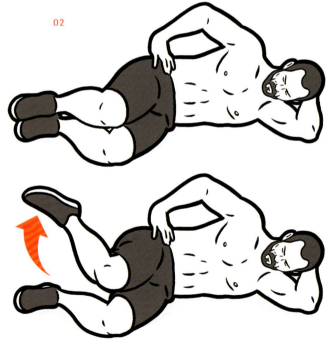

02

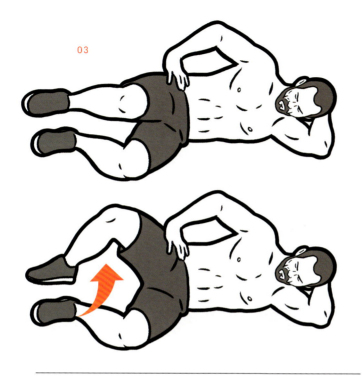

03

03. OPEN CLAMSHELL

▶ Starting from the clamshell position, lift your right leg so that the knee and foot are about 6 inches above your left knee and foot.

▶ While keeping your right foot still, raise your right knee. Hold for 3 seconds, then close your right leg and lower it to the starting position.

04. OPEN REVERSE CLAMSHELL

▶ Starting from the open clamshell position, keep your right knee in place while raising your top foot. Hold for 3 seconds, then close your right leg and lower it to the starting position.

05. HIP EXTENSION WITH ROTATION

▶ Starting from the open clamshell position, extend your right leg behind you, keeping it parallel to the ground. Your right knee should remain flexed. Raise your right foot, hold for 3 seconds, then lower it to touch the ground.

04

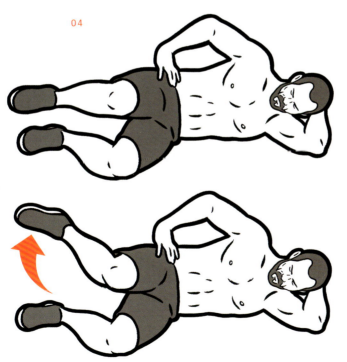

05

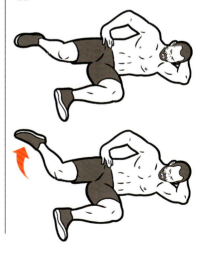

TOTAL BODY

Now that you know how to stretch your hips, shoulders, and spine, you have just one order of business left: You need to put things together. Truth be told, your hips, shoulders, and spine all work as a unit during every moment of every day (and during every single exercise, too). Play tag with your kids, and your hip mobility may help you change direction—but only if your spine delivers proper rigidity. And your hips, spine, and shoulders work together to help you hold your infant in one hand a cup of coffee in the other.

So yes, you should stretch all those joint groups together, too. And that's what you'll do in these final two stretches. Perform 2 sets of each of these each way at least 2 times per week.

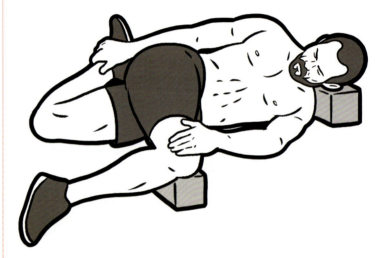

BRETTZEL 1.0

▶ Lie on your left side with your head supported on a foam roller (a rolled towel also works) and place another support under your right knee. Your hips should be stacked on top of each other. Bend your left knee so it forms a 90-degree angle.

▶ Using your left hand, grab the back of your right knee and with your right hand, grab the ankle of your left foot. (If you can't reach your ankle, use an extension strap.)

▶ Take a deep breath, then exhale and rotate your shoulders away from the right knee as far as possible so that your face is looking at the ceiling or as far toward your right shoulder as possible.

▶ Take three deep breaths in this position. Return to the starting position. Do this for two more 3-breath cycles.

▶ Adjust your body so that you're lying on your right side and will be rotating left. Repeat the movement for three 3-breath cycles.

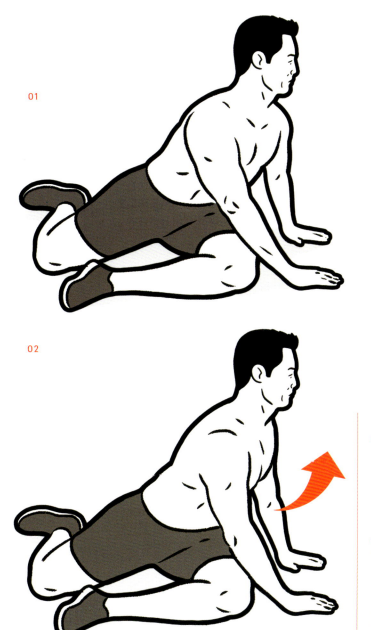

01

02

BRETTZEL 2.0

▶ Start from a sitting position and shift your weight to your left side. Next, bend your left leg so it forms a 90-degree angle with your hip and stretch your right leg behind you. Then, bend your right knee so that your leg forms another 90-degree angle (1).

▶ Rotate your torso to the left (2). Put your left elbow and forearm on the ground. They should be roughly in line with your hips and pelvis. If you can, try to put your right forearm on the ground as well. The goal is to position your shoulders parallel to your left thigh.

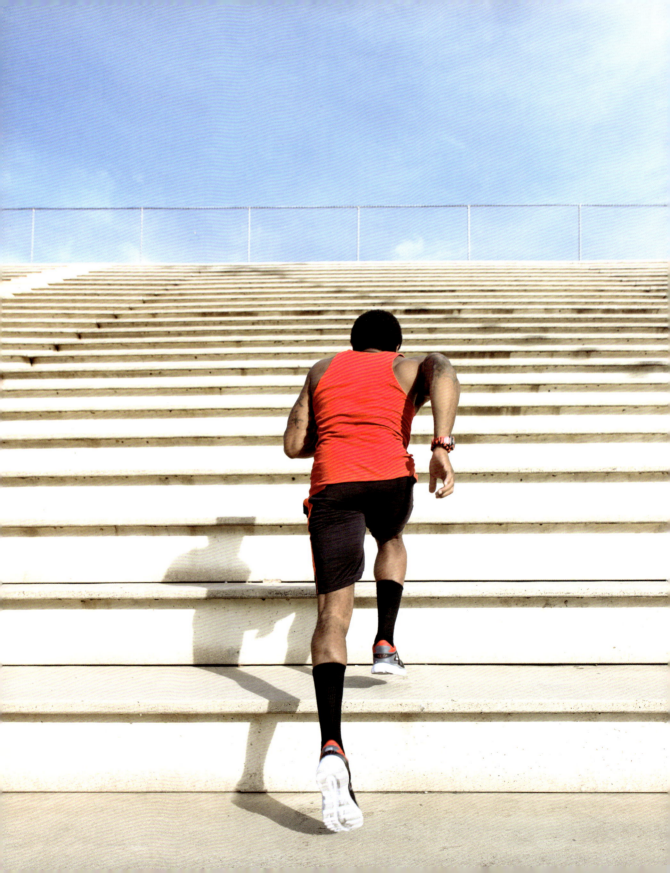

CHAPTER

06

SUPERCHARGE
YOUR ENERGY

IN THIS CHAPTER, YOU'LL...

LEARN TO REBOOT YOUR ENERGY—EVEN ON YOUR MOST SLUGGISH DAYS

CUT THROUGH THE HYPE AND PICK RECOVERY PRODUCTS THAT DO WHAT THEY SAY

STOP WASTING TIME ON SUPPLEMENTS AND TOOLS THAT DON'T WORK

YOU WAKE up early. When you roll over to get out of bed, you feel so sore from yesterday's lift that you want to stay put. Why are you so sore? And so quickly? Then you remember your lackluster recovery routine. And that you're supposed to be at the gym in an hour. Why'd you agree to meet so early today?

You drag yourself to the bathroom, stubbing your toe along the way. You put toothpaste on the toothbrush and promptly drop it on the floor. You think, "Damn, it's going to be one of those days." It's inevitable. You were tired after working late yesterday and didn't go to the grocery store. So, no egg white scramble this morning. You trudge through an uninspiring workout and a workday that devolves from tedious to unproductive.

This is the fourth time you've felt like this in two weeks. You wonder if this is what your 40s are going to be like. You know you need something to boost your energy and mood. That soreness is getting ridiculous. You need to level up in that department as well.

Dude, I feel you. We've all been there. Those days suck. You're in a rut and can't find the energy to get out. If you're like me, even the smell of coffee gives you a headache. No pick-me-up there.

You think more about the dizzying number of supplements available. What's good? What's garbage? Recovery gear isn't any easier. From vibrating foam rollers to cryotherapy chambers to infrared rooms, it seems like something new is coming out every other day.

But you're not getting any younger. You need to level the playing field now. Supplementing your diet plan and cleaning up your recovery process is a must.

There are more than 120 million internet hits when you search for energy- and immunity-boosting supplements and for exercise and athletic recovery gear. That's a lot of reading and watching in order to research what works. Most guys won't look at more than a few sites. How do you know what's good? I'm the nerd who has looked at a lot, experimented a lot, and used a lot—and here are my suggestions.

SUPPLEMENTS

Worldwide, the nutritional supplement industry is supposed to reach $505 billion in sales by 2028. And each of those companies is telling you how much you need their products. They're trying to convince you that their products will help you. When you were in your 20s, you kind of believed them.

And somehow, they're even more convincing now. They spend a few billion of those dollars to study you and your psychology. You are still susceptible to their advertising. They've learned they get a rise out of you by hitting you where it matters most.

You want the daily energy, stamina, and quality workouts you had 15 years ago—or even better. But what do you buy, and is it more than placebo? What does science say?

What To Try

As I've said before, I'm not the biggest supplement person. That's partly because the word "supplement" means "in addition to" not "instead of," and that's something a lot of people forget. But many of you only have time for a processed shake instead of eight ounces of cooked chicken.

I also have serious trust issues. Companies want your money and won't hesitate to lie to get it. I've seen countless ads that claim a supplement has "natural" ingredients, but there's not a single natural food listed on the jar.

The US Congress passed the Dietary Supplement Health and Education Act of 1994 to regulate dietary supplements. At that time, there were only about 4,000 supplements on the market. Now there are more

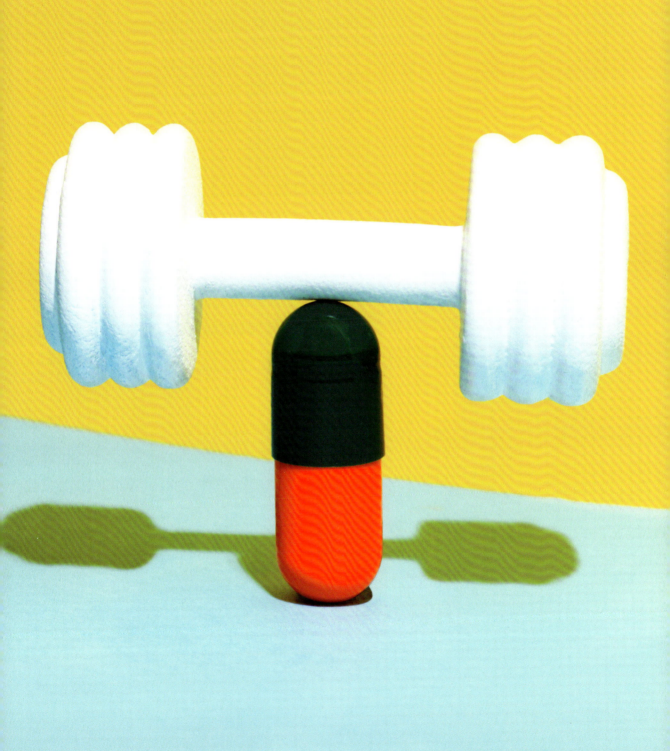

than 50,000, and more than a thousand more are introduced every year. That growing number makes enforcement of the regulation nearly impossible. However, there are some that have proven their value time and time again. Here are a few I've found that are worth trying.

▶ ASHWAGANDHA

From the management of stress to the reduction of blood sugar levels to the reduction of symptoms of depression, this root may have almost as many benefits as cannabis.

START WITH: 2,850 mg daily

▶ CREATINE

If you are trying to build muscle or maintain muscle, get this stuff. It may be the most researched weightlifting supplement that's not a steroid. It works. Also, creatine is not just a supplement for working out. It also helps battle depression. Multiple studies that have shown the benefits of creatine for brain function.

START WITH: 3-5 g daily for building muscle

▶ FISH OIL

I attended a lecture given by nutritionist Robert Yang, who happens to be a colleague of mine. He showed a slide that featured a picture of his son drinking fish oil from the bottle.

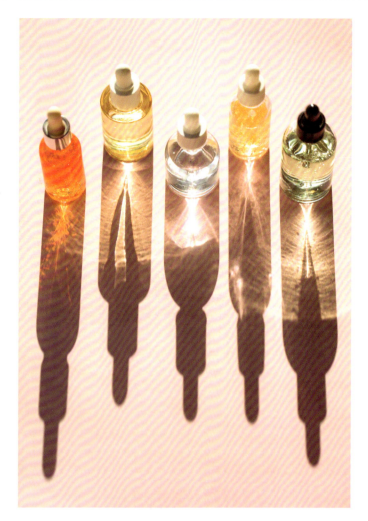

Robert made a joke about it, saying it was one of his proudest moments as a father. I thought it looked disgusting, but I laughed. I also bought a bottle of fish oil. I take a couple of tablespoons a day to make sure I get a few more omega-3s, which help reduce muscle inflammation, swelling, and stiffness.

START WITH: 3,600 mg daily

▶ THC/CBD

People have been using the cannabis plant for thousands of years with amazing health benefits; some that you might enjoy are reduced stress, anxiety, and pain. There is ample research to back up the medicinal claims.

START WITH: 10 g THC and 10 g CBD for sleep; 500 mg CBD daily

▶ VITAMIN D

With the right conditions—such as living in sunny, cloud-free San Diego—this supplementation is not needed. Go outside. Soak in the sun. In the wrong conditions—such as living in gloomy, snowy, Syracuse, New York, or eating an incomplete diet—you need to have this supplement on hand. START WITH: 600 IU of vitamin D2 and D3 daily

▶ WHEY PROTEIN

This is the only supplement on this list I do not take; I tend to get protein from foods such as turkey, chicken, beef, pork, eggs, and more. But I cannot argue against its efficacy—research shows that it works. It's easy to store. It's quick to make. It's also one of the cheaper supplements to get, based on volume. START WITH: 2.2 g protein per kilogram of bodyweight daily

What To Skip

I won't tell you not to take a particular supplement because I have no clue how your body chemistry will react to whatever it is you're taking.

But the placebo effect is real. You can build an entire ecosystem around your weight loss, fat loss, muscle gain, weight gain, immunity boosting –or any change you're trying to make. For example, you want to lose

body fat, so you're eating better and at the right times. You're working out for fat loss. You're sleeping better. You're hydrating more. You have effectively done everything you need to do to increase the potential and possibility for fat loss.

Then you drink that Super Duper Thermal FAT BURNER! Or pop a few fat-burner pills. Voilà, you start losing body fat. Must be the Super Duper, right?

You know you've done that. Or you know somebody who has done it and swears by the supplement instead of looking at the environment for success that was created. I'm not trying to throw too much shade. But these are some supplements that I suggest you use with caution.

▶ VITAMIN C

You start to get that telltale itch in the back of your throat, and odds are good that you'll be pulling out the vitamin C and oranges. But research has yet to prove that more vitamin C is better or that it adds a layer of protection against the common cold. Nothing has proven that it shortens the length of cold symptoms, either. The Centers for Disease Control recommends you get 1.5 to 2 cups of fruit a day and 2 to 3 cups of vegetables. Eat right and you will get more than enough of this vitamin.

▶ CALCIUM

This is the "bones and brains" supplement. As you get older, your body removes more bone than it makes, especially if you lead a sedentary lifestyle. Likewise, your nervous system function slows. Calcium helps both of these. But, as with other vitamins, more than adequate amounts of calcium can be found in a solid diet. There is even research that suggests calcium supplements increase the risk of cardiovascular diseases and heart attacks in men. Add salmon, kale, broccoli, arugula, and collard greens to your diet instead of taking this supplement.

▶ GLUCOSAMINE AND CHONDROITIN

It's amazing how popular these are with the over-40 crowd. They supposedly help with arthritis and joint pain. Science doesn't agree. One meta-analysis (an investigation of multiple studies) found that the combination of the two fared no better than a placebo in alleviating pain. Another study had to be halted because the test group (given a combination of the two supplements) actually started feeling more pain than the group given the placebo.

▶ **FAT BURNERS. SEXUAL-PERFORMANCE SUPPLEMENTS. TESTOSTERONE BOOSTERS**

It's very easy to lump all of these together. They're all jokes. I shouldn't have to say anything about these. But I get questions about them all the time. Fellas, get more sleep. Hydrate better. Exercise more, including lifting more heavy weight. Work on reducing the stress in your life. Stop watching all that porn! If none of that helps, then go see the doctor.

SUPPLEMENTS: THE BOTTOM LINE

At the end of the day, supplements are all about experimenting. We all have different body chemistry. You have to figure out what works for you. The most important thing about that experimentation is giving your body and mind a chance for success. But before you try anything: Clean up your diet. Hydrate well. Exercise. If you still feel like something is missing, then it's time to look for the proper supplement.

RECOVERY GEAR

Much like the supplement industry, there are so many modalities for recovery on the market that it's difficult to figure out what works and what doesn't work. Every advertisement touts a product's ability to help your joints and muscles repair and recover faster than everything else on the market.

Each company claims its tech is the latest and greatest thing, and each company may be right. The problem: science is unable to keep up with the amount of technology being introduced. Either that, or the science is commissioned by the companies who make the technology.

There is also an interesting dynamic in the "feel good" factor. That means if something is helping you recover or makes your joints feel better, you'll think it's the right product. Look no further than professional baseball for a good example of this. Numerous studies show that swinging a weighted bat in the on-deck circle leads to a slower swing speed at the plate. Yet an overwhelming number of baseball players do this every time at bat because it makes the bat feel lighter and they feel better at the plate. With that in mind, I won't tell you what tools I think aren't worth your time. If it makes you feel amazing, go for it. What I will tell you about are the recovery tools that have helped me bounce back between workouts faster and with more energy.

▶ **FOAM ROLLER**

I have soft foam rollers, hard foam rollers, and vibrating foam rollers. I've given foam rollers for birthdays and holiday gifts. Yep, I like the foam roller a lot. I was late to the foam roller magic—I didn't start using them until after I turned 40. I found that delayed onset muscle soreness (DOMS) gets seriously intense after 40. Either that, or my tolerance for pain decreased drastically. But the foam roller has been a godsend for my muscle soreness and my joint range of motion. Everybody who comes to The Playground learns how to use it. There have been zero complaints. I spend a minimum of 5 to 10 minutes a day on a roller.

▶ **MASSAGE GUNS, E-STIM, AND TRACKERS**

Even if you're old-school about your workouts, it's worth introducing some tech into your recovery routine. I have a couple of massage guns that help my muscles get going even after my toughest workouts. I got my first one in 2018 after being a part of a demonstration. The first time it hit my calf was an ah-ha moment. I didn't know if it worked for range of motion, but it felt great on my muscles. I bought it and began using it daily. Then I started hearing chatter from movement specialists about it being a novelty device and about how the sensations are false positives. Then

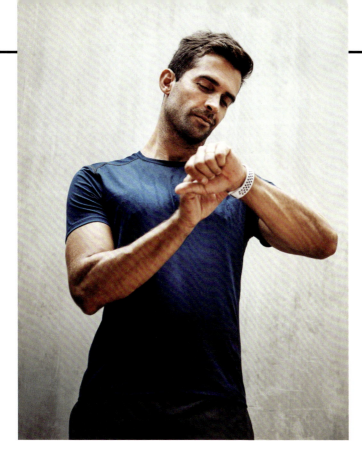

strain I am ready to put on my body for the day. I don't always listen to its suggestions, but it does give me a heads-up on how my day might go energy-wise. And that insight can help me level my expectations.

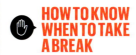

HOW TO KNOW WHEN TO TAKE A BREAK

BELIEVE IT OR NOT, part of being unstoppable is knowing when to stop. This couldn't be more true than in the case of tired muscles. For most of us, next-day soreness is part of hitting the gym. It's technically known as delayed onset muscle soreness (DOMS), but you may know it as that aching sensation that makes walking up the stairs after leg day feel impossible. It's part of the muscle breakdown process. When you put stress on your muscles, it results in micro-tears, which cause inflammation. This can cause DOMS. It often occurs 24 to 48 hours after your gym session. It's tempting to push through it and hit the weights again, but that can actually lead to more pain. Continuing to work those sore muscles can increase your risk of injury, further delaying your gym time. Instead, focus on recovery and consider the tools mentioned in this chapter.

I read more about whole-body vibration therapy and targeted vibration therapy. It's used to improve bone mineral density and quality of life for people living with Parkinson's disease. Even NASA was looking at vibration therapy to mitigate muscle and bone loss in astronauts. More than anything, though, it makes me feel amazing.

You might have seen electronic stimulation (E-stim) units at your physical therapist's office. These tools send mild electrical pulses through the skin to help stimulate muscle fibers or manipulate nerves to help reduce pain. The stimulation of the muscle fiber causes it to contract. The contraction improves blood flow, which helps the repair process. I use E-stim tools after workouts in which I'm reaching 80 to 100 percent of my 1-rep max, and I notice a difference in my recovery.

Finally, consider giving a fitness tracker a try. Think of it as a recovery barometer. The device can help you gauge how your body is responding to your workout, and what you need to do to fully restore your energy. Mine gives me a data-driven idea of how rested and recovered my body is, how much sleep I need, and how much

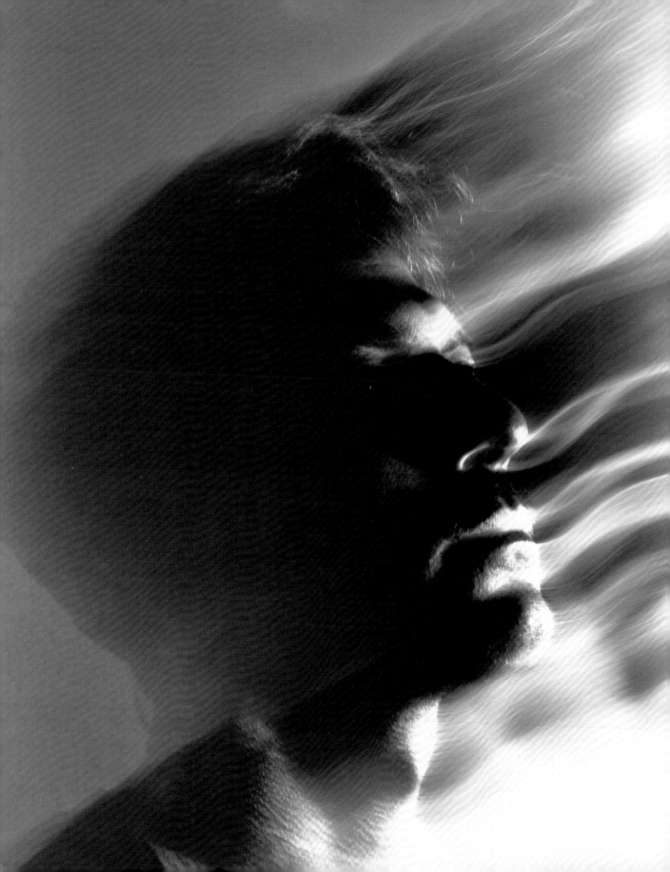

CHAPTER

07

IN THIS CHAPTER, YOU'LL...

LEARN THE FOUR
ELEMENTS OF
BECOMING MENTALLY
TOUGH

HANDLE SETBACKS
WITHOUT LOSING
MOTIVATION

BUILD A GAME PLAN
FOR LIFE AFTER 40
AND BEYOND

BUILD AN UNSTOPPABLE MINDSET

WE'VE SPENT the last few chapters talking almost exclusively about your over-40 body and how we can strengthen it. But one of your greatest weapons after age 40 is your mind—and cultivating a strong mindset can help you overcome many of the challenges you're dealing with.

That's something I frequently work on with my male clients. As a life coach, I'm trained to help people focus on what matters to them and how they can take steps to reach their goals. I partner with men over 40 to deal with what's happening in their lives right now and to help them focus on their relationship with their own lives and on how they can direct it productively through obstacles and setbacks.

And these obstacles run the gamut. They can include everything from athletic setbacks and relationship issues to self-improvement, with things like building confidence and developing tools to stand up for their convictions.

Take Jennings (not his real name), for instance. He was a confident, assertive, and proud person in every way but one. Jennings was terrified of public speaking or even speaking to groups of strangers larger than a few people. It affected his work in a major way. He was an integral part of several teams, but never a team leader—

though he had been asked to take that role many times. He feared losing his job. That is, until he followed the principles outlined in this chapter. He shifted his mindset and eventually earned multiple promotions because he was able to give presentations that landed high-value business for his company. Over time, you can work to build a mindset that is limitless and unstoppable—and this will carry you to success.

My goal in this chapter is to give you the tools that will help you rewire your mind, the most pliable and powerful organ you have. It will help you carefully evaluate any situation by understanding where you are presently, and this will kickstart a transformative process that enables you to unblock your thinking and realize powerful ways of being. You'll be able to accomplish goals you've had for a long time.

This powerful new mindset will invigorate your body more than you expect. Living an unstoppable lifestyle is proactive and fluid, constantly changing and adapting. It's a long-term endeavor. It is holding true to your fundamental beliefs, so you do not succumb to trends and fads, yet also keeping your mind open to exploring new possibilities and opportunities.

FOUR STEPS TO AN UNSTOPPABLE MINDSET

Whenever you're struggling through a problem (and I know these can pile up because of work worries and home issues and gym struggles, among other things), turn to this simple and effective method I developed to help my clients and myself work through setbacks and challenges. I call it Limitless Logic. It's a four-step approach that helps you realize your boundless potential in every situation. I've used this workhorse of a tool often over the past 15 years, sometimes multiple times a day.

Build it into your own mental algorithm, and use it when you're facing a challenge at work, pondering the start of a new business, or trying to figure out your next gym goal.

It will prevent you from ruminating on the negatives, help you open your eyes to the reality of a situation, and give yourself a plan to move forward. Rip these pages out and keep them in your back jeans pocket for a few days. You'll thank me. And now, here's your four-step process.

I. Assess What's Really Going On

Before you even consider what you should do, step back and evaluate where you are and what kind of challenge is in front of you. Enter this process with a full understanding that you may be delving into multiple areas simultaneously. This also forces you to stare your challenge in the face instead of avoiding it.

Like the physical assessment from Chapter 2, this is the most important aspect of creating a mindset that allows you to handle any issue. It's your foundation. And like certain aspects of the fitness assessment, parts of this can feel excruciating. I've been there. I've looked at myself in the mirror and known that I wasn't feeling as happy as I used to feel or that I screwed something up. Sometimes I had to realize that I just needed to accept my situation and that my involvement in it was real.

The challenge you're facing might be mental, physical, emotional, social, or spiritual. Ignoring it or hoping it goes away will only magnify the issue, because you'll be wasting time and not moving yourself forward. To help you give the challenge at hand an honest assessment, answer these questions:

What emotions am I currently feeling about this situation? Describe them.

_____
_____
_____
_____

What do these emotions say about the person I am?

_____
_____
_____

Is what the emotions say fact or interpretation? Use the "cup test" to distinguish between fact and interpretation. Can you get a cup of it? You can get a cup of water or grapes. But can you get a cup of loser or a cup of failure?

_____
_____
_____

Are your interpretations empowering or disempowering?

_____
_____
_____

For each disempowering interpretation, what is an empowering scenario you can create?

_____
_____
_____
_____

Here's an example of what your answers might look like:

What emotions am I currently feeling about this situation? Describe them.
I'm frustrated that I had to cut my workout short because of my back pain. Part of me is angry. Part of me is sad. Part of me simply doesn't understand how I hurt myself—I do these lifts all the time.

What do these emotions say about the person I am?
I'm incompetent. A failure. I'll never measure up to my brother.

Is what the emotions say fact or interpretation?
Incompetent = interpretation
Failure = interpretation
Measuring up = interpretation

Are your interpretations empowering or disempowering?
Incompetent = disempowering
Failure = disempowering
Measuring up = disempowering

For each disempowering interpretation, what is an empowering scenario you can create?
Incompetent—I am disciplined about my gym routine. What new exercises can I try to alleviate my back pain?
Failure—I can't be a failure if my back pain was caused by exercising. At least I'm not sitting on the couch all day.
Measuring up —This is an opportunity I can use to practice more patience. What tools do I have for that?

2. Identify Your Ultimate Goal

Now that you know where you stand, put that in the larger context of what you want in life. Don't get caught up in the immediate outcome of the situation. Sure, maybe you didn't achieve your goal of mastering that new lift, but was that your big-picture goal? Or was it something larger, like staying strong and energized so you can chase your kids around? Maybe it was something less tangible, like making your family proud. Whatever it may be, focus on that and the sting of the current challenge will fade.

If you're not sure what that ultimate goal is, answer this question: if you couldn't fail, what do you want to happen in this situation?

Don't worry about being realistic here like you were in Step 1. Realism kills possibility. Think seriously about the perfect outcome for the situation.

Whatever happened to lead you to this point was the onset of the issue. This stage is how you choose to respond. Maybe you had no part in creating the situation you're working on. After all, you didn't decide to strain your back. Or maybe you are somewhat responsible for this situation, because you skipped your warm-up. Either way, you have the ability to choose how

you respond. Your choice goes a long way toward dictating your attitude and temperament throughout the process.

Pick a lackluster outcome and the energy that goes toward that result will be anemic at best. But if you choose the perfect outcome or most exciting possibility, or even something that seems impossible, your energy and your approach will be much more robust. Try it now.

If I couldn't fail, what would I want to happen in this situation?

_____
_____
_____
_____
_____
_____

Example:
If I knew I absolutely would not fail, I would keep working out to lose that weight I put on last year. Then I'd have more energy to play games with my kids after work.

3. Make a Plan

You're over 40 now, so you're wise enough to know that throwing the proverbial crap against the wall and hoping it sticks rarely works. You need to plan how you're going to deal with this issue. The size and depth of the issue doesn't matter. Make. A. Plan.

The smaller the issue, the smaller the plan. The more intense the issue, the more intense the plan should be. But either way, keep the plan as

simple as possible. You might naturally go for the more complex approach. But your brain works better with small chunks of duties.

If you realize in Step 2 that your ultimate goal is to keep up with your kids, your plan to lose those 10 pounds and gain more energy might look like this:

▶ **Step 1: Knowledge.**
Find out what I know and, more importantly, what I don't know. Learn new exercises that won't aggravate my back pain.

▶ **Step 2: Roadmap.**
Plan your workouts. Figure out what you're going to do and on what days. Put it on your calendar.

▶ **Step 3: Experience. Consistency.**
Bring discipline to this new gym routine. It's the day-to-day execution of the plan hat will make it successful.

▶ **Step 4: Evaluation.**
Assess your progress. Find out what's working and what's not. Make changes accordingly until you find the sweet spot.

4. Ask for Help

Don't do this solo! I am definitely guilty of refusing assistance when facing a challenge. I used to think, _Help? What the hell is that?_

Trust is something I have worked on a lot. I've forced myself, kicking and screaming, to a point where I feel comfortable asking for help and knowing that the help is genuine.

But mastering the ability to ask for help is critical to any good plan. Doing so will let you leverage your best skills and abilities, while relying on others who have better skills in areas that you don't.

It also makes the issue real: You have to share it with somebody instead of keeping your thoughts to yourself. And it's not nearly as hard as you think.

You: Hey, Ivan, I really need some help with this.
Ivan: Ok. What do we need to do?

No need for long, drawn-out explanations. Just ask. We not-so-simply need to find a way to trust. That trust is not only in others. That trust is in ourselves as well. We must trust and have confidence that we have the ability to pick the right people to help us.

I can't urge you enough to use this tool. It may seem a bit hokey at first. But its power lies in forcing you to take an honest look at yourself and responding accordingly. In the next few pages, I'll show you how to put this process into action with real-life examples of challenges you might encounter.

HOW TO HANDLE
COMMON SETBACKS

EXTENDED WORKOUT HIATUSES AND UNEXPECTED INJURIES HAPPEN TO THE BEST OF US. BUT IF YOU FACE THEM WITH THE RIGHT MINDSET, THEY DON'T HAVE TO PUT YOUR PROGRESS ON PAUSE.

EVEN THOUGH 40 is just a number, it can still mess with your mind. For some of us, 40 is midlife crisis time.

But what if turning 40 wasn't a crisis? What if it was a wake-up call, alerting us to all the important things we have left to accomplish?

That was what happened to me. When I turned 40, I realized that I still had a lot of work to do. If anything, turning 40 made me more motivated than ever.

In addition to training athletes, I became a life coach and organized retreats for business and community leaders, started a long-term athletic development program for children as young as 2 years old, and got involved with diversity programs.

But I couldn't have done this unless I had a strong mindset. Here are a few mental setbacks that I've seen—and experienced—in my life, and how to cope with them.

THE PROBLEM:
YOU CAN'T TRAIN BECAUSE YOU INJURED YOURSELF ON A "BASIC" EXERCISE.

First, put the injury in perspective. Blew out your shoulder? You can do lower-body and core work until it heals. Sprained an ankle? You can do upper-body exercises. Unless I'm in serious pain or a workout could cause more damage, I never make excuses. You shouldn't either.

Next, find out what you did wrong. Poor mechanics? Weak stabilizer muscles? Talk to a trainer, a physical therapist, or even a friend. Once you find out what you have done wrong, you can avoid doing it again in the future.

THE PROBLEM:
YOU TOOK A BREAK AND NOW YOUR WORKOUTS ARE REALLY HARD.

You're never going to feel successful if you have unrealistic expectations—and expect-

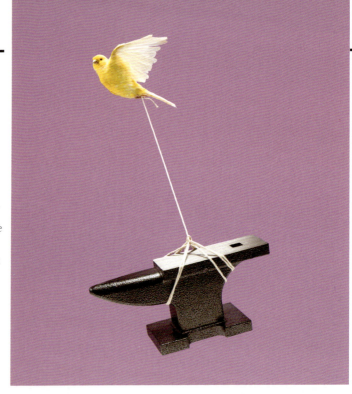

ing your fitness levels to stay the same after taking a break is unrealistic. (Sorry, but it's true.) It takes consistent work to maintain your strength and endurance levels. I've said it before, but it bears repeating: If you don't use it, you lose it. Make a plan for progress and give yourself some time to work back to your former level.

THE PROBLEM:
EVERYTHING WAS EASIER 10 YEARS AGO.

Are you sure everything was easier when you were younger? It might have just been youthful overconfidence. Regardless, it comes back to expectations. You need to do something 3,000 times (the right way) for it to become a habit. That takes time. If you haven't done a particular movement for years, it's no surprise that you're not executing the exercise perfectly. Find a trainer who can help you learn new moves and improve your old ones.

THE PROBLEM:
YOU'RE STRUGGLING TO BATTLE THROUGH A NAGGING INJURY.

About a year ago, I took a spill on my mountain bike and messed up my hip pretty good. And I didn't go to the gym and chase PRs the next day. I called a team of professionals to help

me recover. But all too often, I see people pushing through the pain to finish a squat or a deadlift, contorting their bodies into positions no one should ever be in. Folks, if something hurts, don't ignore it. Find someone who can help you. From there, make a plan. Once you have a roadmap to recovery, you'll feel a lot more optimistic.

THE PROBLEM:
YOUR MOTIVATION IS WEAK.

Let me guess—when you were young, you wanted a six-pack and bulging biceps. And that's what I wanted, too. But now that we're over 40, we don't feel the need to check our physique in

the mirror every 15 minutes. (That's what I like to call progress, by the way.) I say the same thing to everyone who walks into my gym—don't tell me what you want to look like or what your goal weight is. Tell me what you want to do. Your goal shouldn't be to lose 10 pounds. A much better goal is to hike up to the top of, say, Pike's Peak. When you're doing what you love—surfing, golfing, chasing your kids around the backyard (anything but jogging, really)—yes, you're going to get in better shape, but you're also going to feel a lot more confident about yourself. And confidence is something that's really attractive.

MY BEST ADVICE:
40-YEAR-EDITION

I'VE LEARNED A LOT IN THE 50 YEARS OF MY LIFE. HERE ARE THE TIPS, TRICKS, AND ADVICE THAT HAVE CHANGED ME FOR THE BETTER.

▶ **BEST WAY TO SQUEEZE IN A WORKOUT:** Schedule it. Being a trainer doesn't mean that I prioritize exercise over everything else. (Hey, I have other things going on, too.) In the past, I used to fit in a workout whenever I could, but life often got in the way. Scheduling my workouts is the only way to make sure I follow through on them. Never end a workout without determining when your next one will be.

▶ **BEST WAY TO FIND DOWN-TIME:** Schedule that, too! Even blocking off a few hours a day helps. On days when I feel overwhelmed, I really look forward to doing nothing.

▶ **BEST PROFESSIONAL ADVICE:** Learn to say no. I was always that guy who was helping out with other people's programs. Once I started saying no, I was finally able to prioritize my own goals.

▶ **BEST WAY TO SLEEP:** I sometimes struggle to get 7 to 9 hours of sleep, so I started focusing on my sleep quality instead of sleep quantity. I have a fitness tracker and its algorithm tracks my sleep efficiency. One thing that helps: I never go to bed hungry or thirsty. And because I need some white noise and air circulation, I use a fan year-round and have some music playing. Keeping a dark bedroom also helps.

▶ **BEST STRESS RELIEVER:** Cut down your debt. I'm not rich. Never have been. But once I started chipping away at my debt, I felt a lot less stressed.

▶ **BEST WAY TO UNWIND:** Watch a comedy. I love laughter, and I love comedy that's genuine and unfiltered. Good comedians are a godsend.

▶ **BEST ADDITION TO YOUR DIET:** Berries. For years, my fruit intake was pretty limited, but once I expanded my diet to include blueberries, blackberries, and raspberries, I also started feeling healthier overall. Maybe it's all the antioxidants.

▶ **BEST WAY TO SAFEGUARD YOUR MENTAL HEALTH:** Let it go. I'm almost ashamed to admit it, but I used to hold grudges. Now that I've learned to move on, life is much easier.

My ultimate advice? Keep going. Keep moving. Never slow down. The momentum you built with this book will serve you decades from now so you can truly remain unstoppable, no matter what comes your way.

THANK YOU

For Purchasing
Unstoppable After 40

Boost your fitness with more from *Men's Health*.
Visit our online store and save **20% off your next purchase.**

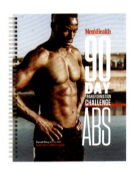 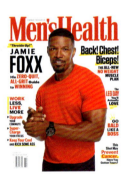 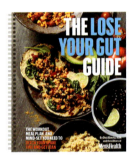